The Dad's PLAYBOOK
TO LABOR *and* BIRTH

The Dad's PLAYBOOK

TO LABOR and BIRTH

A PRACTICAL AND STRATEGIC GUIDE TO PREPARING FOR THE BIG DAY

THERESA and BRAD HALVORSEN

THE HARVARD COMMON PRESS

Boston, Massachusetts

The Harvard Common Press
535 Albany Street
Boston, Massachusetts 02118
www.harvardcommonpress.com

Printed in the United States
Printed on acid free paper

Library of Congress Cataloging-in-Publication Data
Halvorsen, Theresa
   The dad's playbook to labor and birth / Theresa and Brad Halvorsen.
      p. cm.
   Includes index.
   ISBN 978-1-55832-672-9 (pbk. : alk. paper)
   1. Labor (Obstetrics) 2. Childbirth. 3. Fathers. I. Halvorsen, Brad. II. Title.
   RG652.T44 2012
   618.4--dc23
                                        2011025959

Special bulk-order discounts are available on this and other Harvard Common Press books. Companies and organizations may purchase books for premiums or resale, or may arrange a custom edition, by contacting the Marketing Director at the address above.

Book design by Elizabeth Van Itallie

Cover photograph by Lynn Parkes

Interior photographs, p. vi: ©iStockphoto.com/DirKaDirKa; p. viii: ©iStockphoto.com/Martine Doucet; p. xiv: ©iStockphoto.com/nyul; p. 30: ©iStockphoto.com/Linda Kloosterhof; p. 44: ©iStockphoto.com/Piotr Marcinski; p. 60: ©iStockphoto.com/Rich Legg; p. 92: ©iStockphoto.com/Terri Hutchison; p. 114: ©iStockphoto.com/Steve Goodwin; p. 148: ©iStockphoto.com/RonTech 2000

Football art: ©GettyImages/Scott Heiner

10 9 8 7 6 5 4 3 2

Theresa would like to dedicate this book to her friend Taryn, who took the time to explain what a doula was and then held Theresa's hand (metaphorically) during her first few births. Without Taryn's passion for childbirth and parenting, Theresa wouldn't have become a doula, childbirth educator, prenatal yoga instructor, and parenting writer—she'd probably be miserable in a cubicle somewhere. She thanks Brad, who always supported her crazy ideas, one of which was this book. She'd also like to thank all the men who shared their birth experiences with her, her former doula clients from whom she learned so much, and the thousands of parents who inspired her with their questions and their own passion about birth and parenting. She's grateful to the other birth professionals in the Sacramento area for their support and to her parents for their support and love. Finally, she'd also like to dedicate this book to her sons, who put up with their crazy mom and her crazy ideas. Without them, she wouldn't be in this field.

Brad would like to dedicate this book to Theresa, with thanks for introducing him to a field he knew nothing about when they first met. He also would like to thank her for their interesting dinner conversations, which would disgust other people. Finally, he would like to say thanks to his family and his kids for keeping life entertaining.

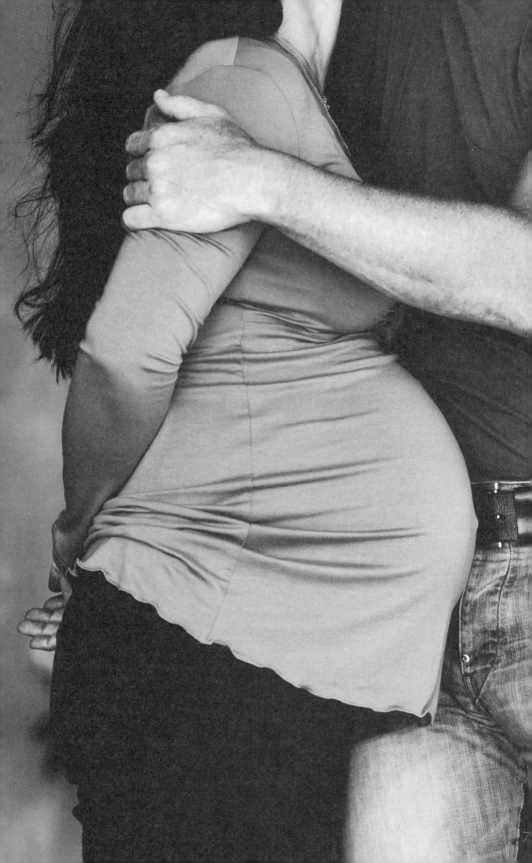

Contents

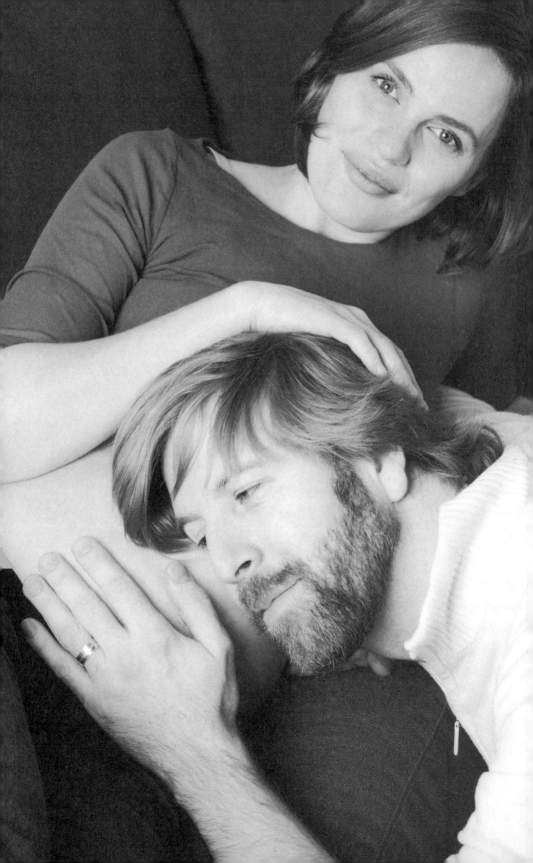

Introduction
Why Are You Holding This Book?

You're holding this book because your partner is pregnant and now everyone expects you to be her "coach" during labor. Judging from the stories you've heard from your friends, coaching is more than showing up on the big day, holding her hand, and giving her ice chips. You're holding this book because you want to do everything in your power to make the birth of your child as perfect as possible for you and your partner, whether she's planning on getting an epidural or aiming for an unmedicated birth.

Let's start with some scenarios just in case you're not yet convinced that you need this book.

Scenario I

You're at home and your partner's having pretty strong contractions. You've called the hospital thinking it's time, but the nurse said it's not; the contractions aren't close enough together yet. The nurse wants the two of you to stay at home for now. But your partner is complaining about how much the contractions hurt and asking for help. What do you do?

Unless your doctor or midwife tells you otherwise, you'll be at home in early labor with a woman who is experiencing potentially curse-inducing contractions until the contractions are "strong enough" and "close enough together" to head to the hospital. Although the contractions aren't yet as bad as they're going to be, many women need a lot of help from their coaches during this part of labor. After thinking long and hard, you realize you can't get your partner an epidural while you're still at home. This means you are her epidural. It means you have to know how to help her during these hours at home.

Scenario 2

You just got to the hospital. Your partner's contractions are strong. Verbally, she has gone from uttering an occasional swear word to acting like she's starring in a Kevin Smith movie. She is threatening you, the admitting nurse, and the doctor she hasn't even seen with bodily harm if these contractions don't get easier. Her head is about to whirl around 360 degrees, and she's going to puke green vomit at any second. The very nice, calm nurse has assured the two of you that your partner will be getting an epidural "soon." Two hours later, you're still wondering where the epidural is.

In many hospitals, an hour or even two may pass from the time a woman walks through the door in labor until she gets relief from an epidural. Hospitals have procedures regarding the use and administration of epidural medication; these procedures are meant to keep Mom and the baby safe. Until your partner can get the epidural, you have to help her. You have to know what to do. You have to have a playbook.

Scenario 3

Your partner really wants to go unmedicated; she wants to avoid an epidural at all costs. She's relying on you to help. She's already told you that if she asks for an epidural your job is to say no. Now you're wondering how on Earth you're going to tell this woman you adore, who is about to be in a great deal of pain, that she can't have medication.

Maybe a part of you is wondering whether it's truly possible for your partner to go unmedicated. It *is* possible—if she has a strong, knowledgeable coach. She's really going to need you. You have to know how to help her.

Scenario 4

Your partner has gotten the epidural, and everyone has just breathed a sigh of relief. She is back to her charming and beautiful self. Now you're thinking that the work's over and you can sit back and get some sleep.

Unfortunately, you're wrong. Although you may have less to do after your partner gets an epidural, you still have to help her. An epidural controls pain by numbing a person from the waist down, making the belly, lower back, legs, and hips numb. So your partner is going to need your help in turning from side to side and getting comfortable. And, because she's numb, she may have more trouble pushing the baby out, so you may have to give her extra help at that point, too (see page 115).

Here's another thing about epidurals. Most anesthesiologists agree that, even when epidurals work the way they're supposed to, they take away only 70 to 80 percent of a laboring woman's discomfort. Whereas some women find they're very comfortable after getting an epidural, others still need to use coping techniques like controlled breathing and massage.

And, yes, sometimes an epidural simply doesn't work the way it is supposed to. Think about dental work. You probably know someone who has difficulty getting numb enough for fillings. You probably know someone else who gets completely numb from a single shot of novocaine and stays numb for several hours. Everyone responds differently to medication, and some women don't respond well to an epidural. So, after your partner's epidural she may find she's not numb from the waist down, or at least not as numb as she expected.

Are you starting to understand why you're holding this book?

Now, why does all this matter? Because her experience of the birth will shape your future together as a family. Women who are unhappy with the way their babies' births went have a higher chance of getting postpartum depression. And a woman's partner is a big factor in her satisfaction with her birth experience. So, the better a coach you are, the less likely your partner will be unhappy with the experience and the less likely she'll have postpartum depression.

Trust us: You really don't want your partner to have postpartum depression. Not only is a woman with postpartum depression just plain miserable, but she may not bond with her baby, her baby's growth and development may be delayed, and she may struggle in her relationship with her partner.

Still not convinced you need this book? Here's one more reason.

Many men say they'll do anything their partners ask during labor. All the woman has to do is ask. Then Dad's surprised when Mom asks for nothing in labor. He's even more surprised when she's pissed at him afterward for not helping during the birth. What did he miss?

Women often don't ask for things they need during labor. It's like the connection between her mouth and brain is broken. Why is this? Think about what you're like when you've hurt yourself badly. Are you thinking clearly? Are you able to tell other people what to do to help you? Now think how you are when you're angry, sad, or scared. Are you thinking clearly then? Are you able to give detailed instructions about ways to make you feel better? Now, combine being in a great deal of pain with feeling angry, sad, or scared, and you have an idea of what your partner may experience during labor. She's incapable of telling you what to do. It's your job to know what to do to help; it's your job to read her mind.

Helping a woman in labor is like coaching a kids' soccer team. If you know nothing about soccer, you can't do as good a job as coach. You'll do a better job if you take a seminar about coaching soccer to kids. Think of this book as that seminar.

We've broken up this book into easy-to-read, easy-to-skim sections. Although we recommend reading the book from beginning to end, you should feel free to skip around. We've tried to make it easy for you to get the information you need so you can be the best coach you can be. If you come upon a term you don't understand, check "Birth Jargon Explained," which begins on page 162.

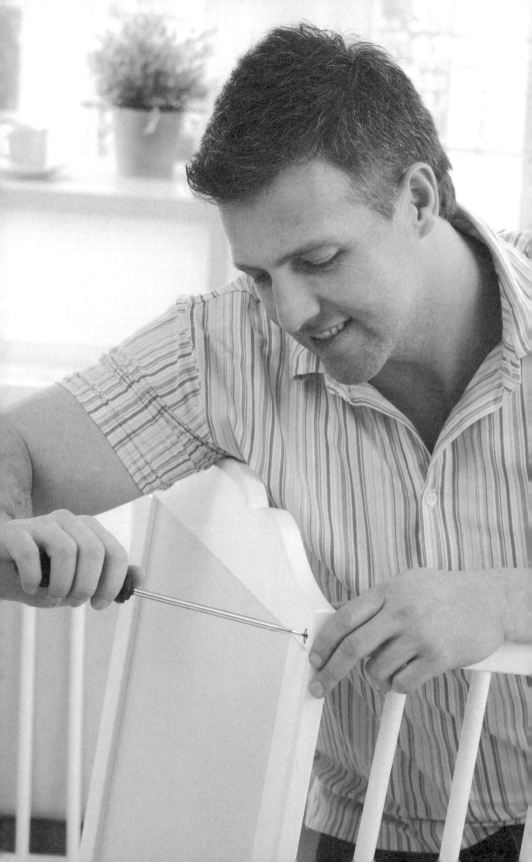

Chapter 1

YOU'RE GOING TO HAVE A BABY!

Time to Get Ready

ou've noticed a transformation in your partner over the past few months. Her body is changing. A lot. And we have an important tip about that. Don't call attention to her appearance with cute little pet names, like Orca (Brad's brainchild), or you may never hear the end of it (right, Brad?).

Both of you are starting to think about the big day, the birth of your baby. Your partner is talking on and on about birth plans, what happened in a television birth she watched, and the horror stories about birth she's heard from friends and family members. If you've gone along on at least a few prenatal appointments, you are getting to know the doctor or midwife and getting some questions answered. You may have signed up for childbirth classes, in which you will see videos showing not only women's private parts but babies coming out of them, too. You've painted the baby's room and filled it with overpriced furniture. Maybe you've started worrying about sleepless nights and mountains of baby poop, or anticipating the tax deduction your child will bring. You've imagined playing catch with your kid or holding out your pinky while sipping pretend tea.

But are you prepared for the actual birth?

Back in the day, women relied on other women in the community to help them have their babies. As the dad, you would have gone out to hunt or farm, or paced in circles around a fire, or your guy friends would have taken you out to get hammered. Your grandfather and maybe even your father sat in a waiting room and passed out cigars when the nurse came running in to say that the baby had been born. But those days are gone. Now you have to be there at your baby's birth. And you can't just show up; you're the coach.

Think about labor as the Big Game. It lasts only an hour or two, but the team spends many more hours preparing for it, physically and mentally. And the better the team does at practices, the better the game goes. Labor is a lot like that. It lasts for only a few hours, or maybe a whole day, but for it to go as smoothly as possible you have to prepare for it.

So this chapter is all about prep work. You'll find out what your partner wants for the birth and what you should expect from her during labor, depending on her personality. You'll learn about the classes you should take and about choosing other people to support her—and you—at the birth.

Talk to Your Partner

The first thing you have to do is talk to your partner to determine what her goals are for this birth. Maybe she wants to go epidural-free, or maybe she wants you to book an anesthesiologist to come to the house and give her an epidural at the first hint of pain (which wouldn't be possible no matter how much money you offered). Maybe you've taken a childbirth class together and your mind is full of ideas about massage, breathing techniques, positions, and visualizations. Maybe your partner has enrolled the two of you in a HypnoBirthing class, or maybe she's been bouncing around the house on a birthing ball. In any case, you have to know her wishes so you can support her to the best of your abilities.

You have an advantage over the nurses, midwife or doctor, and other helpers at your baby's birth: You know your partner better. You know when she's ready to explode in anger like a nuclear bomb, you know when she's ready to burst into tears, and you know how to help in both situations (yes, you do, or she wouldn't still be with you). You know her moods and her wants. You have many ways of knowing the things she'll prefer during labor.

But modern birth can involve unusual decision making. If you're going to advocate for your partner in whatever circumstances may arise, you have to talk with her about her preferences ahead of time. Between baby showers, work, and other obligations, we know, it can be hard to find time to talk. If necessary, schedule a meeting to have this conversation! When the time comes, turn off your phones, the television, and other distracting devices.

Be prepared for her to avoid the subject of the birth; a lot of pregnant women are in denial about the fact that they're about to pop out a baby. Even if your partner is eager to talk, you will probably need multiple conversations to find out what you need to know to support her. She may change her mind regarding procedures such as the epidural after taking a class and maybe even during labor. Keep communicating, and try to be flexible.

Take time to explore your own feelings about birth and babies, too. Are you excited, or does the thought of birth make you queasy? Do you have any wishes for the birth other than a healthy baby and a healthy mom? Do you secretly hope, for example, that your partner will get an epidural and squeeze this baby out within an hour? Or are you concerned about the potential side effects of medications? Are you hoping she'll have a cesarean so you won't have to see her in pain? In any case, you need to process your own thoughts. Her body is hers, but she is your partner, and the baby belongs to both of you.

Consider Her Personality

Your partner's personality helps determine how she processes information and responds to situations. Understanding her personality can help you figure out what will help her in labor and what won't. It will help you know how to talk to her during labor, not to the anonymous laboring woman you learn about in childbirth class.

Dr. Jekyll or Ms. Hyde Although generally a woman's personality can tell you how to support her during labor, your partner may surprise you. The quietest women can become the noisiest during labor, and vice versa. Occasionally the nicest, calmest, gentlest personality can transform into a megabitch.

Introvert or Extrovert?

The most important distinction regarding your partner's personality is whether she's an introvert or extrovert. Introverts, on the one hand, tend to be private and reserved. They need a lot of time to themselves; interacting too much with other people can drain their energy. They rejuvenate themselves in isolation or in silence. Extroverts, on the other hand, tend to be outgoing and enthusiastic. They feel energized when they're interacting with people and drained when they're alone. Since opposites attract, your partner may want the opposite of what you'd want. It's important to be aware of this, because labor is all about her.

You know your partner is an introvert if

— She prefers quiet,

— She becomes overwhelmed in noisy situations,

— She gets tired after spending time with a lot of people or in noisy situations,

— She usually doesn't listen to music in the car or while working, especially if she is stressed,

— She enjoys staying in after a long, hard day, and

— She's more of a listener than a talker.

She's an extrovert if

— She's very sociable,

— She enjoys going out with groups and talking with friends on the phone,

— She feels energized after loud or people-filled activities,

— She likes a party or a night out on the town after a busy day,

— She likes being the center of attention, and

— She always has music playing, the TV on, or people around her.

Not everybody fits the label of introvert or extrovert, but most people lean in one direction or the other. Now, how does this relate to labor?

Introverts in labor. Introverts often want their labors to be as quiet as possible. If your partner is an introvert, she may want silence in the room. She'll want the lights dimmed. She may deal with contractions by moving to a quiet spot, shutting her eyes, and focusing inward. She'll probably want you close by, but she may not want much other help from you.

Introverts are easily overstimulated, so silence the phone, and keep the number of people in the room to a minimum. Discourage friends and family from popping in to say hi. Try to minimize the staff in attendance, and avoid having nursing or medical students in the room, if possible. For more advice about managing support people, see page 66.

Extroverts in labor. Extroverts are people people. If your partner is an extrovert, she'll probably want many people around her in labor, to help or just to say hi. She'll likely be chatty during early labor and may enjoy playing games (pack some playing cards!). She'll find loud, energetic music and talking to be welcome distractions. She may even agree that your cheesy jokes are hilarious. Extroverts often enjoy having the spotlight on them even during labor, so your partner may become annoyed if not everyone is focused on her. She also may have difficulty figuring out whom she wants in the room when the baby is ready to come out.

What if your partner is in the middle of the range from extrovert to introvert? Flexibility is the key with this personality. Perhaps your partner will want one or two extra people in the room, but not a lot. Maybe she'll like music during labor, but only if it's soft and gentle.

SCENARIOS TO CONSIDER

If you're a planner by nature, you may feel better if you know ahead of time what you would do in the situations described as follows. Talk through possible responses with your partner.

• What if your partner calls you at work to say that she is in labor?

• What if you're someplace where your partner can't reach you?

• What if her labor is very long?

• What if she yells at you while she's in labor (see page 89)? What if she cries?

• What if you feel that nothing you do is helping?

• What if she wanted an unmedicated birth but is starting to change her mind in the middle of labor? (Talk about every medical intervention that she wants to avoid, especially if she wants to go unmedicated. Learn techniques to decrease the need for common interventions, and talk about what you will do if the intervention seems truly necessary.)

Perhaps she'll like the room dim, but not dark. Make sure you talk with her about her wishes during labor and be prepared to turn the music off or on and to kick people out if necessary.

How Does She Make Decisions?

Many people can make good decisions quickly, but others need time to think things over. For example, when shopping for shoes (we know, you try to avoid going along whenever possible), does your partner ask to try on one or two pairs and then make a quick decision? Or does she try on a dozen pairs, become distracted by a stunning pair of sandals (even though it's December), try on each pair of shoes multiple times,

----

• What if the birth ends in a c-section? (See page 111.)

• What if you get sick or injure yourself during labor? Who will come to help your partner?

• What if she can't use the pain-relief measures of her choice? For example, what if your partner wants to walk the halls and labor in the shower, but the doctor won't let her out of bed (see page 107)? What if you've both planned to use massage during labor, but she finds that she hates it? What if she wants an epidural but learns that it's too late to get one?

• What if the people whom your partner doesn't want in the room show up anyway? Or if someone whom your partner has chosen as a helper turns out to be unhelpful? (See page 67.)

• What if neither of you like a particular nurse, doctor, or midwife? Does your hospital allow a change? (See page 70 for advice about firing a nurse.)

• What if the baby has to go to the neonatal intensive-care unit (NICU) immediately after birth?

gradually reduce her pile of possibilities to six pairs, wonder if she can find them online for a better price, call her sister to ask, put the six pairs on hold, and then try on another dozen? If so, she needs time to process information before making decisions.

The way your partner makes decisions can affect her birth experience. Let's say the doctor comes into the room and offers to break the bag of waters (this procedure is called an amniotomy; see page 110). The mom who makes decisions quickly will say yes or no. The other type of mom needs time to think things over. Here's why.

Women who feel that they had no control over the way they gave birth, that they didn't get time to make decisions regarding their care or didn't receive all the information they needed—especially if the birth didn't go well—are often traumatized by the experience. They may have recurring negative thoughts about the experience or about birth in general, and even, in rare cases, nightmares. Studies have found that these women are more likely than other mothers to experience postpartum depression.

If you know that your partner is slow to make decisions, talk with her about common obstetric procedures before she goes into labor. Plan to give her time during labor to make non-emergency decisions. Always remember, if staff members are *asking* whether they can perform some intervention, there is no emergency. Your partner can take a few minutes to ask questions, get answers, and make a good decision.

How Does She Handle Pain and Stress?

In general, the ways your partner handles pain in daily life can give you an indication of how she'll handle labor. The things she does to ease her pain and stress in other situations will probably help her in labor, too.

For example, does she love water? Does she take multiple showers a day or climb into the bathtub after a hard day? If so, the shower or bath may be helpful for her during labor. Does she like getting a massage? Does she like to go for a long walk when she's stressed? If yes, then guess what? You've just figured out other ways to help her in labor. Have her tell you her top five ways of dealing with pain and stress, and you've just found your top five ways to help her during labor.

Here are some more tips. If she paces when stressed, she may like moving around during labor. If she lies in a dark, quiet room when stressed, she may want darkness and quiet during labor. If she yells and throws things when in pain, guess what she's going to do during labor?

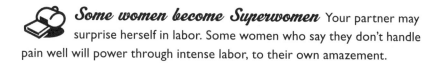 **Some women become Superwomen** Your partner may surprise herself in labor. Some women who say they don't handle pain well will power through intense labor, to their own amazement.

Although we will briefly discuss some of the pros and cons of obstetric procedures such as the epidural, this book is about how to support your partner whether or not she uses such technology. (For detailed information about medications and medical procedures in childbirth, consult one of the many books on the subject, take a childbirth class, or talk with your doula or your partner's doctor or midwife.) Following is a list of other, more low-tech things that your partner may find helpful in labor. Discuss them with her, your childbirth educator, the doctor or midwife, and any friend or relative who will be helping at the birth. If your partner really wants something special, like a birthing tub, check to make sure your hospital will allow it.

HYDROTHERAPY (WATER)
— Shower
— Bathtub or birthing tub

SOUNDS

— Listening to music

— Moaning, chanting, singing, or humming

— Praying

— Talking

VISUAL AIDS

— Dim lights

— Focal point (see page 74)

— Closed eyes

— TV or movies

TOUCH

— Hugs

— Massage (hand, foot, back and shoulder, head and face, or belly; see page 11)

— Cool compresses

— Warm compresses or heating pads

— Ice packs

BREATHING (see page 80)

— Slow breathing

— Patterned breathing (hee-hee-hee-blow)

POSITION AND MOVEMENT

— Walking

— Slow dancing or swaying

— Rocking in a rocking chair

— Using a birthing ball (page 163)

— Assuming positions such as standing, sitting, on hands and knees, and kneeling

MASSAGE FOR LABOR

Most women find that massage helps them a great deal during labor. As with everything else in labor, though, there are things to try and things to avoid. Here are some tips.

- **Find out what kind of massage she likes.** If she prefers foot rubs over hand rubs, chances are that'll hold true in labor. Does she like a lot of pressure or just a little? Does she like you to rub or press vigorously with your thumb or palm, or does she prefer a more gentle massage? Would she like having her belly rubbed?

- **Plan on massaging her back.** Most women love having their backs rubbed during labor, for hours and hours and hours and. . . .

  When you're giving a back massage, in general you want to start at the top, work downward, take your hands off, and then start at the top again. Rubbing up and down the back or arms is annoying. Pretend she's a cat: If you ruffle her fur, you'll get scratched.

  If she has back labor, a special kind of back massage will be vital. See page 100.

- **Try hand massage.** An epidural may require ten to twenty minutes to take effect, and even after that the medication may be less effective than your partner would like. Instead of throwing up your hands in despair, you can give her a hand massage to help her get through the contractions. (For more advice about what to do if an epidural doesn't work, see page 108.)

- **Use massage oil.** A massage lasting only a few minutes doesn't require a lubricating oil. After a few minutes of rubbing, though, your hands and her skin will get chafed. Oil can keep this from happening. Many women like a floral- or citrus-scented massage oil in labor, but others find such smells overwhelming. To be safe, bring along both scented and unscented oil. Lotion can substitute for massage oil if you reapply it often.

MISCELLANEOUS

— Visualization or meditation (see page 171)

— Self-hypnosis

— You! Never underestimate the power of your presence.

If She Wants to Avoid an Epidural

Many women want to avoid an epidural during labor for a variety of reasons, including the potential side effects spelled out in the sidebar. If your partner wants to go unmedicated, there are some extra preparations the two of you should take:

Take a childbirth class geared for couples who want to go unmedicated.

Talk with your partner's doctor or midwife. Many care providers are very supportive of couples who want to go unmedicated. Others aren't. The rates of epidurals and cesareans among a provider's clientele can tell you a lot. So can the induction rate, because inducing labor—forcing it to begin—can lead to a more difficult labor, which can increase the need for an epidural and the odds of a cesarean. If your partner's provider seems unsupportive of natural birth, a switch may be in order.

Decide what you'll do if your partner asks for an epidural during labor. Does she want you to talk her out of it? Should you wait until she asks three times? Does she want to choose a code word that will mean she really, really wants an epidural?

PROS AND CONS OF EPIDURALS

PROS

• Epidurals are usually effective at relieving pain.

• They allow a woman to push.

• Mom gets a chance to rest before pushing the baby out.

• Little of the medication reaches the baby.

• The medication doesn't knock a woman out or even make her drowsy.

CONS

• The woman cannot be upright, and lying down can interfere with the progress of labor.

• The slowing of labor increases the likelihood of other interventions, such as the use of Pitocin (see page 169) and an amniotomy (see page 110).

• The pain relief may not be as great as expected (see page 108).

• The mother's blood pressure may drop, and this can affect the flow of blood through the placenta to the baby.

• Because of the risk of a drop in blood pressure, the mother has to wear a blood-pressure cuff. The cuff squeezes her arm every fifteen minutes. This can prevent her from getting needed sleep.

• The mother may shiver, itch, feel nauseated, vomit, and run a fever.

• Pushing is more difficult, because the woman's pushing muscles are numbed. This increases the chances that a vacuum or forceps (see page 119) will be needed to get the baby out.

• The mother may be more likely to struggle with breastfeeding during the first few days after birth. (There's a great deal of conflicting information about this side effect, which lactation consultants don't yet fully understand.)

- There is a small chance that the epidural will cause a headache and backache a day or two (and sometimes for longer) afterward.

- Actually getting the epidural may be unpleasant. To place an epidural, the anesthesiologist will request that Mom sit still for several minutes, and this can be very, very difficult during contractions.

- New studies show that women are often frustrated by the lack of support, help, and attention from the support team after an epidural.

Take Some Classes

Your partner has just come home from one of her prenatal appointments with a long list of classes available for pregnant couples. Besides childbirth classes, there may be baby classes, breastfeeding classes, anesthesia classes, cesarean classes, sibling classes, early- and mid- and late-pregnancy classes, car-seat classes, and safety classes. You imagine your weekends and evenings disappearing—before the baby even arrives.

How many of these classes are actually necessary? Not all of them, fortunately. Read the course descriptions carefully, and ask what the doctor or midwife recommends. Some of the classes will overlap. Hospital tours (see page 16) may be included in some but not in others. You may be able to choose between a weekend childbirth course and one that's spread over several weeks; you're not expected to take both.

If you're still confused, you or your partner should speak to someone who teaches the classes or is in charge of the curriculum. This person can consider your plans for the birth and let you know which classes will help you most and which you can consider extra.

It may occur to you that your partner's the one who needs to take these classes; you can opt out of some of them, right? Sorry, but that's wrong. You need to go along to get your own questions answered

WHICH IS BETTER—A PRIVATE OR HOSPITAL-BASED CLASS?

Theresa, who has taught both private and hospital-based classes, feels that they each have pluses and minuses. Sometimes hospital educators are limited in what they can say about birth, the doctors, and the facility. Hospital-based classes tend to be biased in favor of epidurals, partially because most of the women who take hospital-based classes want epidurals. On the plus side, hospital-based classes are usually cheaper and easier to find than private classes. In addition, the hospital teacher knows a great deal about the hospital's policies and may let students know which ones can be bent (Theresa always does—don't tell her supervisor!). These classes usually follow a Lamaze or ICEA curriculum (see page 173), though Lamaze and ICEA classes are also taught privately.

Private classes are great for couples hoping for unmedicated births. The instructors are often certified by organizations such as Bradley or HypnoBirthing (see page 172), in which case they teach specific theories and comfort techniques. In a private class, you may learn about less mainstream ideas such as using cloth diapers, making your own baby products, and "green" parenting (avoiding chemicals). Private courses often are longer, and so allow more time for getting to know the other couples. Some private classes include art, journaling, meditation, or even drumming circles.

and to absorb some of the information that your partner (who has pregnancy brain) may miss. This means you even have to go to the breastfeeding class. In leading such classes, Theresa teaches dads what a "proper latch" looks like (moms have a hard time judging from the pictures, because they look down at their boobs rather than straight at them) and how to help their partners with breastfeeding during the first couple of weeks.

Do the costs put you off? If you truly can't afford the classes you and your partner want to take, talk to someone at the birthing facility or, if you're considering private classes, speak to the instructor. You may be able to arrange for a decreased rate or payment over time.

Don't put off signing up. If childbirth courses run for six weeks, you can't call when your partner is thirty-four weeks pregnant and expect to complete one in time. In many hospitals, courses fill up two to three months in advance. You or your partner should start calling about classes during her second trimester.

Consider taking some classes after the baby comes. For instance, you might take baby-care and baby-safety classes when you have a real baby to work with. Remember, though, that after the baby comes you'll be busier than ever and sleep-deprived, too. Use caution in planning to take any classes after the birth.

Take a Tour

Especially if you don't get around to taking a childbirth class, be sure to take a tour of the birthing facility. Ask a lot of questions, like these:

— Is a refrigerator, pantry, and ice machine available? Where?

— What are the policies regarding visitors? Does Dad have to leave after the baby is born (see page 132)?

— Do the rooms have chairs or couches for dads or other support people to sleep on?

— Can you tape a picture to the wall, to serve as a focal point during labor (see page 74)?

— Do the rooms have CD players, TVs, DVD players, and MP3 player docks? Is Wi-Fi available and free?

— How do you page the nurse?

— How do you raise or lower the head of the bed?

— Is there a bar at the end of the bed that your partner can hang on to if she wants to squat for the delivery?

— Is a shower or tub available, or both? Are women allowed to give birth in the tub, or is it for labor only?

— What else is available for the laboring woman? Beverages, towels, a birthing ball?

— Where is the thermostat, and are you allowed to adjust it?

— Are there policies about taking still pictures or videos of the birth?

— Will your partner be moved to a different room after the birth? If so, can you see that room, too?

— If there is a high chance that your baby will end up in the NICU (for instance, in the case of twins or triplets), can you see it ahead of time?

— What are the security policies before and after the baby is born?

— Are there forms to fill out ahead of time, like the birth plan (see page 33)?

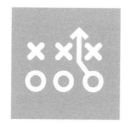

Decide Whether to Use Other Support People

So, your partner is thinking of inviting her mom, her best friend, her sister, her coworker, and that nice lady down the street (whose name she doesn't even know) to the birth. The list of people who are going to see your partner's privates on the big day is growing longer and longer. You imagine visitors standing in the hallway craning their necks as if they're at a rock concert, only instead of trying to see the band they want to see your partner give birth.

Fortunately, the hospital may not allow such a long guest list. Some hospitals limit the number of people in the room during labor, and many limit the number of people present during the actual birth. (There may also be rules about the number of visitors after the baby is born; be sure to check.)

But almost all hospitals allow women to have at least two helpers— Dad included—and many allow more. There are advantages and disadvantages to having extra support people.

Advantages of Extra Support People

Your partner may have an easier labor with extra support. For example, one person can help her with her breathing or hug her while another person massages her back. Or your partner can get foot and hand massages at the same time.

Having another helper takes the pressure off you. It's hard to learn all about birth and comfort techniques in just a few weeks or months—and then to remember everything when the big day comes. (Quick—name three ways to help with back labor. See page 98 if you're stumped.) When you think back to the video you saw in birthing class, you may clearly remember only your reaction to seeing a baby being squeezed out. If someone else is there to help throughout labor, the pressure is off you to remember everything.

You can get some sleep or rest. Once the baby's born, the early days of bonding with the baby and transitioning into being a dad will be one of the best times of your life, an amazing time that you'll remember forever—if you're not completely exhausted. Besides, Mom will still need you to take care of her. Having another helper during labor can keep you from wearing yourself out before the birth.

You can focus on your partner's emotional well-being. You can turn your attention to alleviating your partner's fears and drying any tears while someone else helps her with breathing or position or gives her a massage.

You can deal with your own emotions. Many men push aside their feelings on the big day to keep their partners from seeing how scared or upset or sad (or even exuberant) they are. With someone else in the room, you can deal with your emotions so they don't build up until you have a breakdown.

You can be taken care of, too. Another person can remind you to position yourself comfortably and to eat. You'll feel better about leaving to use the bathroom, get food, or just take a break (see page 63) if someone else will be staying with your partner. You'll be less tired and less likely to injure yourself.

A second person can be really helpful if a c-section becomes necessary. Some hospitals allow only one helper in the operating room, but others allow two. With a c-section, the baby is born very quickly, and then the surgery continues for thirty to forty minutes. If two support people are present, one can focus on Mom while the other focuses on the baby.

If your partner has a cesarean and your hospital allows only one helper in the operating room, ask if a second person can take your place if you accompany the baby to the nursery or NICU.

Disadvantages of Extra Support People

Someone else is there. This other person will be part of the birth story and will thus share a pivotal moment in your lives. You and your partner may want to keep the experience between the two of you. And your partner may not be comfortable exposing herself to another person, even one she knows well.

Your helper may not be helpful. If you and your partner haven't chosen carefully, your helper may drive you both crazy—or, worse, have a bad influence on the birth, your experience of it, and your memories of the event. This leads us to the next section.

Choosing Support People

Say you and your partner have talked it over, and you've decided you want someone else at the birth. How do you choose an assistant coach from among all your friends and family members?

Consider personality. You want someone calming, with a voice your partner likes and a demeanor she finds soothing. Consider your own preferences, too; if you grind your teeth whenever a certain person speaks, she's the wrong one to have at the birth, even if she's assisted at a thousand others.

Make sure your helper can be available. She won't be much help if she can't leave work before five o'clock or find somebody else to pick up her kids. The person you choose should be able to get off work at any time and to easily find someone else to mind her children, if she has any.

Consider what sort of help you want from her. Theresa remembers a couple whose friend was supposed to know everything about birth. They were excited to have her in attendance, but all she did was stand in the back of the room and complain about being cold and hungry. When you invite someone to help at the birth, we suggest that you tell her what you'd like her to do: Run errands? Give massages? Take photos? Filter out casual visitors? (For advice about kicking out people who aren't being helpful, see page 67.)

Realize that experience can be helpful—or not. Theresa has seen people with little experience of birth turn out to be fantastic coaches. People with more experience can be just as fantastic, but some will bring their own agendas. They may try to "save" your partner based on past birth experiences. Make sure your would-be supporter won't use your baby's birth as a means of processing her own bad feelings.

Make sure your helper won't impose her own wishes. Your partner may be happy to have her best friend with her—until your partner desperately wants an epidural and her best friend desperately tries to talk her out of it. You could end up with the two women crying or screaming at each other while your partner is trying to manage contractions. Avoid inviting anyone who disapproves of your plans if you think she'll try to force her opinions on the two of you.

Decide when you'll want help. Do the two of you want extra support during the labor, during the delivery, or after the baby is born? Talk this over so there will be no confusion. Does your partner really want her father-in-law in the room as she's pushing out the baby or breastfeeding for the first time?

YOU NEED ANOTHER SUPPORT PERSON AT THE BIRTH IF . . .

• Your partner wants one.

• You don't think you'd be comfortable witnessing the birth (see page 27).

• You can't stay awake for twenty-four hours or more. Labor can go on for a very long time—in fact, prodomal labor (see page 101) can last several days.

• You have knee, back, or hand problems that make it hard for you to kneel on the floor or give massages.

• You're worried that you'll faint during the birth. You can read about preventing fainting on page 90, but if you're truly prone to fainting then someone else should be ready to take over coaching duties.

The On-Call Coach

If you're undecided about having another person at the birth, consider choosing an on-call coach. This person has to be willing to drop everything and come, but only if you should decide you need help. This is great insurance in case your partner's labor turns out to be long or difficult.

Dealing with security Many labor-and-delivery units are locked and guarded. If this is the case at your birthing facility, tell your support people that they'll have to bring a picture ID, get a visitor badge, and be buzzed in to get to you and your partner.

The Professional Doula

What the heck is a doula, you ask? She is a trained and experienced labor coach. Usually she's hired by the parents-to-be, though some birthing facilities offer volunteer doulas. A doula is great to have if you know you want a helper, but one more experienced than your friends or family members. A doula can help with breathing and positions, and she may be knowledgeable about special comfort techniques such as aromatherapy, massage, and acupressure. She will probably have given birth herself, so she'll have plenty of sympathy for your partner. Think of a doula as a coach who not only has taken an extra coaching seminar but has coached a lot of teams through winning games. By taking pressure off you, she can help you enjoy the birth a little more.

If you're thinking about hiring a doula, here are some things to do.

Find out if the doula is certified. A certified doula has attended trainings and births and is making the doula business her profession. She'll present a written agreement and tell you clearly what she can and can't provide. See page 172 for some certifying agencies and their websites.

Interview two or more doulas. You want not just certification, training, and experience, but also a good match for your personality and your partner's. If you can't stand a doula's voice or mannerisms, all the training in the world won't make her a good support person for you. Questions like these will help you get to know your prospective doula:

— How did you get started as a doula?

— What are your qualifications? Are you certified? Are you a postpartum or antepartum doula as well as a birth doula? (Postpartum doulas help in the home after the baby is born. Antepartum doulas help in the home before the baby is born, often for women on bed rest.)

— How would you describe your birthing philosophy?

— Can you support our goals for the birth—for example, to get (or avoid) an epidural?

— What do your services cost, and what do they include? When do we pay? Do you know whether our insurance company will cover the cost? Do you have a contract for us to sign?

— When should we call you during labor, and what's the best way to reach you?

— Will a backup doula be available if, when labor begins, you're sick, attending another birth, or unable to come for some other reason?

Make sure she'll help you, not take over your job. Unless you don't want to be the main coach, you should make sure your doula won't nudge you out of the way. Let her know why you're hiring her and how you and your partner envision her helping during the birth.

Find out how she views her role. If your partner wants to give birth in a hospital, your doula shouldn't try to talk her into a home birth. If your partner wants an epidural, your doula should do everything in her power to get her one. A doula should support your wishes even if they go against her personal philosophy about birth.

Understand that the doula won't be in charge. Although having the help of a doula can decrease the likelihood that your partner will need pain medications, forceps or vacuum extraction, or a cesarean, these procedures are sometimes necessary even with the best of help. Because a doula has no medical training, she should always bow to the medical expertise of the doctor or midwife and the nurses. She should not make medical decisions for the two of you.

Children

Kids can be wonderful support people at birth, but they can also make things difficult. Imagine your daughter offering a soft voice, a hand to hold, and a cool compress for her mother in labor. Now imagine your young son getting overwhelmed and throwing a fit while your partner yells in pain. Who would you help first, your son or your partner?

If you're thinking of having your children at the birth, here are some things to do.

Talk to the hospital staff. Find out the policy regarding children at birth. The hospital will probably require that the children be healthy and that they be removed if they create a disturbance.

Talk to your children. Don't assume that your kids do or don't want to be there. If they seem lukewarm, let them know that they don't have to take part.

Take age and maturity into consideration. Most children under five years old wouldn't be comfortable at a birth; the medical equipment, the mess and smells of labor, and the expressions and noises Mom makes might scare them. Remember that young children see their parents as superheroes, so it's hard for them to see Mom looking vulnerable.

Enroll the children in a sibling class. Many birthing facilities offer childbirth classes for kids. Television shows about birth can be helpful, too, provided they show normal, uncomplicated births.

Put another person in charge of the children. You can't support your partner and take care of your children at the same time. Someone else should have the sole job of caring for the kids. This person should be willing to take them out of the room, if necessary, and able to soothe and entertain them.

Give the children the right to leave. Most older children do fine at a birth if they can leave the room whenever they feel like it.

Let the children help as much or as little as they want. They might like to offer their mom sips of water or cool compresses, or they might prefer to just observe.

Use kid-friendly terms when talking about medical interventions. Don't get technical; just explain that the medicine will help Mom or the baby. Understand that needles and other medical instruments can frighten a child.

Place the children carefully for the birth. Consider putting them in a corner where they can watch from a distance. If they want to be closer, put them near Mom's head, not at her feet.

THE KIDS' BIRTHING BAG

If you're going to have kids at the birth, each will need a bag of tricks and treats. Here are some suggestions for what to pack:

- **Snacks such as apples, lunch meat, cheese, and crackers.** Leave out sugary foods; you won't want to deal with sticky messes or hyperactive kids. And don't forget a bottle of water, milk, or apple juice.

- **Things to keep a kid busy.** Books, board games, video games, and a portable DVD player are all good ideas. Coloring books and crayons, pencils, or markers are great distractions, if your kid won't be tempted to use the crayons, pencils, or markers on the wall the second someone's back is turned. Be careful with stickers, too.

- **At least one change of clothes.** A child who is messy or not yet potty-trained may need multiple changes of clothes over the course of labor.

- **Sleep necessities.** If your kids are like ours, they won't sleep without a blanket and a stuffed animal.

What If You Don't Want to Watch the Birth?

If you've been attending childbirth classes, you've probably seen videos of babies coming out of women you don't even know. Seeing your own baby being born may be a magical moment for you. If you're like some men in Theresa's classes, though, at this point you may be worrying that the sight will be traumatizing and disgusting. Maybe you're upset about a previous birth experience and afraid of reliving it. Or maybe you're worried that seeing the baby come out will cause problems in the future, during sex or at other times. Some men are afraid they'll faint, or they just want to maintain the mystery of their partners' privates.

Sometimes it's the woman who doesn't want her partner to see her give birth. She just wants to keep some things to herself.

Whatever your reason, you may be considering leaving the room for your baby's birth. Feel free to go if your partner agrees and the two of you prepare for this. Sit down with your partner and explain your feelings. Perhaps simply talking through them will relieve some of your fears.

Be prepared to compromise. Some women feel very strongly that their partners should be with them through the birth. If your partner really wants you there, maybe you can be in the back of the room with your eyes closed, or you can keep your face near hers instead of down below. For more advice about attending the birth without watching it, see page 117.

Even if your partner says she won't mind your leaving the room, you'll want to avoid leaving her alone with the nurses and the doctor or midwife. She needs a familiar person to help her during one of the biggest moments in her life. Make sure that her mom, her best friend, or a hired doula will be there to hold her leg, refresh her with cool compresses, or offer her a drink.

If you leave, don't go far. Plan to come back as soon as the baby is born. Your partner and your baby will need you.

You might change your mind Some dads who thought they wouldn't want to watch the baby come out get so caught up in the moment that they just have to look. Ask your partner whether she would mind if at the last minute you decided to watch.

Prepare for the Baby

Although this book is mostly about birth, we want to share some tips about things to do ahead of time to help those first few weeks with the new baby go a little smoother.

Figure out who will come to help after the birth, and when. You may have a lot of friends and family members who want to help after the baby's born. If you don't plan ahead, though, they may turn out to be more a curse than a blessing. Talk to each of them about what help you'll need and what they're willing to do. Will they do laundry, run errands, cook, or just hold the baby? You may want to create a schedule so you don't have five people over one day and none the next. If these people are from out of town, where are they going to sleep? Will they stay at your house, where the new baby is up all night while your partner is trying to figure out breastfeeding? And what are these people going to eat? Do they expect you to feed them? Entertain them? It's best to figure out all this stuff before the baby arrives.

Buy baby supplies. Now's the time to stock up on diapers, blankets, clothes, and other baby stuff. Don't get carried away, though; it's impossible to predict all your needs in advance, and you will be able to do some shopping after the baby is born. Even with twins, we found it easy for one person to run to the store to get whatever we needed. Besides, it was nice to get out of the house for a little while.

Figure out both of your work situations. If she's working now, when is she going to go on maternity leave, and for how long? How long a paternity leave are you going to take? See page 39 for more information on paternity leave.

Learn how to care for the baby. Take baby-care and breastfeeding classes before the baby is born, if you can. Ask your friends and family members for advice about caring for a newborn. If your insurance company will allow it, choose a doctor for your baby before the birth. (If your insurance company doesn't allow this, a pediatrician on staff at the hospital will examine your baby after the birth.)

Make sure your chores are done. If there is a home repair or heavy gardening job that needs to be done around the time of the birth, do it now, if possible. This is also a good time to prepare casseroles or other foods to freeze for those days with the new baby when neither of you will feel like cooking.

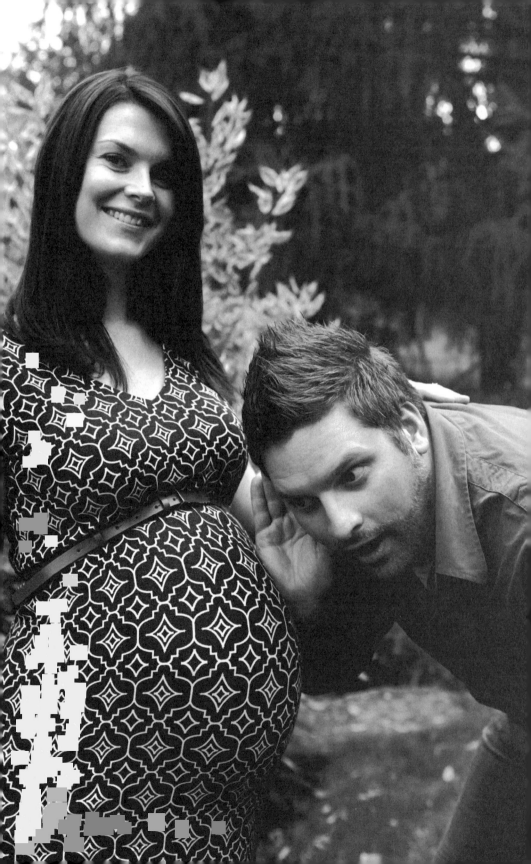

Chapter 2
ANY DAY NOW:
Last-Minute Things to Do

ou're down to the wire. By this point you should know what your partner wants for the birth, and you should have your support people in place. Now it's time for last-minute chores, because the baby is coming in just . . . wait—do you actually know when the baby is coming?

What's Up with the Due Date?

Everyone is asking about your baby's due date, and you're freely giving it out. You may even be saying, "The baby will be born on December 4." But the chance of your partner's delivering on her due date is very low, only 3 to 5 percent. That date is supposed to be forty weeks into the pregnancy, but babies normally make their appearance at any time between thirty-seven and forty-two weeks. This means that your baby can come at any point during a five-week window—if he doesn't decide to arrive early. Even an ultrasound exam can't tell you exactly when the baby's going to come.

How exactly do medical professionals figure the due date? If you went along on the first prenatal appointment, you know that the doctor or midwife asked your partner when her last menstrual period started.

The due date is forty weeks after the first day of the last period (technically, the doctor or midwife identifies the month and day by going back three months from the first day of the last period and then forward seven days).

Are you starting to see a problem with this? The calculation is based on the assumption that every woman has a twenty-eight-day menstrual cycle and ovulates (releases an egg for fertilization) on day 14 of that cycle. In reality, this isn't true. Some women have a twenty-two-day cycle, and other women have a thirty-four-day cycle. Although most women ovulate in the middle of their monthly cycles, some don't. Variations in cycle length and ovulation time are among the reasons that due dates are so inaccurate. We don't know exactly when your partner ovulated, so we don't know when your sperm combined with her egg to make your little spawn.

Another problem may be that your partner's memory isn't accurate. Unless she was tracking her period on a calendar, she may have guessed about the date that her last period started. Her inaccurate memory could add to the inaccuracy of the due date.

What causes labor to begin? We still don't know the answer to this question, but we're pretty sure it's a shift in hormones that starts when the baby's lungs are fully mature. Inducing labor, rather than letting it begin naturally, is risky, because the baby might not be ready to breathe properly. For this reason, many doctors won't induce labor simply for reasons of convenience—that is, just because Mom's tired of being pregnant or because she wants to have the baby before Thanksgiving.

Help Write the Birth Plan

Remember all that talking you did last chapter? Now you and your partner should be writing up all her wishes as a birth plan or wish list. You'll give this document to the medical staff at your birthing facility to help them get to know you, your partner, and her goals for this birth. The birth plan will become part of your partner's medical chart. It will help the staff view you as individuals, not just as another couple having a baby.

Many birthing facilities now have a birth-plan form that they encourage women to use. If you and your partner dislike the form, though, you can substitute your own version, tailored to your needs.

Be flexible. Just because you say you want to avoid a particular medical intervention doesn't mean it won't happen. Sometimes a procedure such as a Pitocin drip (see page 169) or vacuum extraction (see page 119) is necessary to save the life of the mother or baby. Try to avoid the words *no* and *I want*. If you make the nurses pissy, they won't want to help you as much. Instead, write, "We'd like the help of the staff to avoid an episiotomy" or "Laura would like to go unmedicated; we'd appreciate any tips you can offer." The staff will be more likely to help you if you ask them nicely. (For more information about getting what you want out of the hospital staff, see page 68.)

Keep the plan to one sheet. The nurses have a great deal to do, and they're not going to read through a binder full of information about you and your partner. Give them a shorter plan, and they'll be more likely to read it and try to stick to it.

Mention only requests that are unusual or important. You don't need to say that your partner wants music playing or the lights low. It's not the nurses' responsibility to turn on music or dim the lights; it's yours, as the coach. You should, however, specify whether your partner wants an epidural and whether you want to delay newborn procedures (see page 124). If you plan to play a didgeridoo at the birth (one dad did, at a birth Theresa attended), your nurses will want to know that. It's a good idea to include the names of support people, too.

Review the plan with the doctor or midwife before labor begins. Many couples make requests that can't ever be fulfilled at their birthing facilities or that will automatically be denied because of a medical condition. Unless you and your partner go over the birth plan with her care provider, you may be very disappointed on the big day.

Create a Cheat Sheet

How are you going to remember what help she wants from you in labor when you're tired and feeling a little emotional yourself? Create a cheat sheet! Here's where you can remind yourself that she wants the lights dim and music playing, or that she wants to try laboring in the bath. Here are some ideas to guide you as you create your cheat sheet.

K.I.S.S. (Keep it simple, stupid.) Don't bring the entire binder of information from your childbirth class. If your partner hates being touched, you don't need a list of massage techniques, and if your hospital doesn't have a birthing tub, then that information will be useless to you, too. You want only ideas that will help *her*. So modify a few of your class handouts and staple them together, and consider highlighting any medical terminology that might escape you when you're overtired (like "epidural" versus "episiotomy"). Or you might simply make some notes and drawings in a pocket-size notebook. Some dads laminate a single sheet and keep it close by throughout labor.

Have your partner look it over. We know you'll get it right—you're reading this book, after all. But seeing your cheat sheet will make your partner feel better, and she may have ideas of things she'd like you to add. Then put the cheat sheet into your birthing bag (see page 36), because if you arrive at the hospital without your notes, your partner might yell at you.

Get Your Camera Ready

Most couples want pictures of their baby's birth, although opinions about when and what to photograph vary dramatically. The role of photographer, along with so much else, will probably fall to you, so you should keep these guidelines in mind.

Check on hospital policies regarding photography, if you haven't already. Some hospitals will allow still and video photography of anything and everything as long as the birth is going well. Others will allow still pictures, but no videos of the actual birth. Still others won't allow any photography of the actual birth or the moments following it. In the case of a cesarean, most hospitals won't allow video in surgical rooms, and some won't allow still photography, either.

Talk to your partner. Some women don't want any pictures of the labor or birth; they want photos taken only after the baby is born. If your partner does want pictures of labor, should they be PG-rated only, or are NC-17 crotch-shots okay? (If you want a shot of the baby's emergence that doesn't show your partner's privates, try holding the camera by Mom's head rather than over the doctor's or midwife's shoulder.) If your partner is going to breastfeed, will she mind pictures that show her boobs?

Figure out the equipment. Make sure you know how your camera works, how to load a memory card, how to change batteries, and so on. Carry an empty memory card and extra batteries in your birthing bag. Know how best to take pictures in dim light, preferably without a flash.

Plan to take pictures of everything. If your partner doesn't mind, plan to take photos all through the process. You can snap a couple of pictures while you're still at home, a picture of her entering the hospital building, and pictures of the rest of the support team. Remember, though, that taking pictures is always secondary to helping your partner through contractions.

Consider giving someone else the job. When labor gets intense, you'll want to hand the camera to another support person. This way you'll not only be able to devote yourself to helping your partner, but you'll also get to see yourself in some of the pictures later. Or you might appoint someone as photographer for the day. Some couples even hire a professional photographer to take pictures during labor and birth and afterward.

Pack Your Bag

By now, there may be (well, there *should* be) a large bag sitting by your front door, full of clothes, toiletries, and comfort items for your partner and the baby. And your partner may be insisting that you put this bag into the car every time you leave the house.

But is your bag ready? You should have your own, you know, so you won't be digging around in hers to find a snack, and then accidentally pull out her underwear and leave it lying on the floor for everyone to step on. Here's what to pack:

Snacks. They shouldn't have strong odors, and they should be easy to carry. They should provide you with both protein and carbohydrates. Good choices are energy bars, nuts, dried fruit, crackers, and canned or bottled drinks. Use your best judgment when it comes to caffeine. (If you pack an alcoholic drink to celebrate the baby's birth, plan to avoid cracking into it early.) Add a sticky note to remind you to pack a cooler with some perishables at the last minute. They might include non-smelly sandwiches, fresh fruit, and yogurt in a well-sealed container. And don't forget the breath mints.

A change of clothes. Hospitals used to provide scrubs for partners to wear, but now they do this only for c-sections. Not only is it refreshing to change your shirt or pants during a long labor, but birth can be messy, and you may get some of it on you. Besides, if you wear a suit to work and end up going directly from work to the hospital, you could be stuck wearing your suit through the birth. This is how dads get their suits ruined. So bring clothes that will be comfortable for supporting your partner in various positions and for sleeping in. Most dads are comfortable in sweatpants with a T-shirt and sneakers or sandals.

A jacket or a sweatshirt. If labor is long or in the middle of the night, many coaches get cold, no matter what the weather is.

A bathing suit. Many women live in the shower during their labors and like their coaches to be in there with them. Bring your bathing suit so you don't have to go naked. If you do go naked and the nurses catch you, they'll laugh, and for months to come they'll tell stories about that dad who was naked in the shower.

Stuff to keep you busy. If your partner gets an epidural and falls asleep, you'll want to pass the time with a book, magazine, laptop, handheld video-game device, or crossword puzzle.

Medications. If you're on a prescription, don't forget to pack your pills. And bringing allergy or headache medicine might keep you from gritting your teeth or running out to hunt down an open pharmacy.

Cash. It's a good idea to have a few dollars for the cafeteria, vending machine, or parking. Bring one-dollar bills or quarters in case you need to use the vending machine at 2:00 in the morning.

Knee pads. These are handy in case you end up kneeling to give massages for a while. (If you forget your knee pads, a hospital pillow will do.)

BEYOND THE NECESSITIES, FOR MOM

You can make your partner happy by packing some things that she hasn't even thought of:

• **A small, battery-operated fan.** She'll like it even better if it's attached to a squirt bottle (just ask her before you squirt her in the face during a contraction).

• **LED candles.** For mood lighting and focal points.

• **An air-activated heating pad.** Some moms find heat relaxing, and these pads really help for back labor. You can buy one at a pharmacy for a few dollars.

• **Pillows.** Hospital pillows suck! So bring at least one from home. Put an old, colored pillowcase on it so you won't mind getting it dirty and so it won't get mixed up with the hospital pillows.

• **Focal-point picture (see page 74).** A focal point is anything a woman stares at during contractions. Consider bringing a picture you can tape to the wall (if the hospital won't let you tape anything to the wall, put the picture in a frame that you can set on a table). The picture might be of your pet, a place the two of you went on vacation, a relaxing scene, or something funny to make her smile. Some couples use an ultrasound picture of the baby. Talk about possibilities with your partner, or surprise her.

• **Flavored gelatin, frozen juice bars, a sports drink like Gatorade, or a smoothie in a jar.** Your birthing facility may provide such foods for women in labor. If not, a refrigerator-freezer should be available for storing your own. Be aware, though, that some hospitals are still in the Stone Age and allow only ice chips during labor.

• **Flavored syrups for ice chips.**

• **Massage oil—both scented and unscented.**

• **Something to entertain Mom (a magazine or book) or both of you (a game or DVD) in case she gets an epidural.**

- **Recorded music, nature sounds, or white noise.**

- **A birthing ball.** This is the same thing as an exercise ball.

- **Aromatherapy products.** See page 65.

- **A rolling massager, tennis ball, or rolling pin.** This is helpful for back labor (see page 98).

- **Bribes for the staff.** See page 70.

- **Foods she missed during pregnancy.** For example, raw-fish sushi (packed in ice) or unpasteurized cheese. Since these examples are perishable, arrange to have a friend bring them after the birth.

- **A big plastic container.** For the placenta, if you want to take it home (see page 121).

- **Chocolate, flowers, or another special gift for your partner.**

Arrange for Time Off Work

If your partner has a job she wants to go back to, she'll have several weeks to several months off after the birth of your baby. But what about you? How much time do you get off, and is it paid?

Most employers have to follow the federal Family Medical Leave Act (FMLA), though there are exceptions for some businesses. This law says that a father, just like a mother, is entitled to twelve weeks of unpaid leave, and that after this period he can return to the same job or to another with the same pay and benefits. Some states have extended this coverage to employees not covered by FMLA, and some have increased the length of the unpaid leave.

But only a few states offer paid time off. Unless you live in one of these states or your employer offers paid parental leave, you'll be paid only for accumulated sick leave and vacation days.

Find out what your employer offers and how much wiggle room you have. If you're confused, or if the HR person is giving you the runaround, talk to your boss. Do it early; under FMLA, you have to give thirty days' notice before you take your time off. If possible, give your employer even more of a heads-up.

Don't rely on the information your HR person gives you over the phone. Communicate by e-mail, so there will be no confusion about your job situation after the birth of the baby.

Decide when exactly you'll want to be home. Some dads take just a few days off for the birth, go back to work until the friends or relatives have left, and then take some more time off. Others take two full weeks after the birth and then return to work part-time until their vacation or sick leave is used up. This is a good compromise if your employer or your job would suffer without you for several weeks.

Other Things to Do in the Last Weeks of Pregnancy

With every day that goes by, the two of you are a little more excited and anxious. Every morning you wake up wondering if this will be the big day, and every night you go to sleep a little disappointed (or relieved). But the last few weeks of pregnancy can be fun, if you figure out what to do:

Have sex. Unless your partner's doctor told her otherwise, feel free to have plenty of sex. It'll be the last time for a while, so enjoy it; you can't harm the baby. Need another reason? Sexual arousal produces a hormone called oxytocin, which causes contractions. In addition, semen contains prostaglandins, which can "ripen" (soften) your partner's cervix in preparation for labor. If she's not in the mood for intercourse, other things you can do together will provide nearly the same effects. And no, we're not explaining what those things are. Just make it all about her, and you'll do fine.

Stay busy. If you're not going to work, fill your days with chores and fun activities. If you're still working, plan outings for your days off. The two of you won't be alone much longer (assuming you are now), so enjoy your time together as a couple.

Encourage your partner to stay busy. Have her plan something fun to do every day for a week after her due date—lunch out, a shopping trip, a pedicure, a massage, a day trip that keeps her close to town. If the baby's late, these outings may get expensive, but they will help preserve her mental health, and that's priceless. She won't mind waking up each morning to find that labor still hasn't begun, because she'll have other plans for the day.

Install the baby's car seat. All states have laws requiring newborns to be buckled into safety seats before they can leave the hospital. A nurse will probably walk out to the car with you to make sure the baby gets buckled in safely (though she probably won't check to make sure the car seat is properly installed). You won't want to keep the nurse, your partner, and the baby waiting while you try to install the seat at the last minute. It's best, anyway, to have a trained person check the installation. Many insurance companies and fire and police departments will install or check car seats for free, and some baby stores provide weekend car-seat installation clinics. You should also practice clicking the car seat in and out of the base a few times until you feel comfortable with it.

Stay in Touch

In the weeks leading up to labor, many coaches worry they'll miss the big day. With modern technology, though, there's little chance of that unless you leave town. Here are ways to make sure the whole birth team stays connected:

Make a list of important phone numbers. Include the doctor or midwife, the hospital, other labor-support people, and so on. If you have other kids, don't forget to include the number of whoever will be taking care of them while you're at the hospital. Put the list on the fridge if you're still using a land line.

Include extra phone numbers. List your coworkers' extensions, so other people can track you down if your cell phone isn't working. Tell your partner how to reach your company's switchboard operator, who may be able to locate you if no one else can.

Program important numbers into your cell phone and your partner's.

Carry your cell phone at all times. If your company doesn't allow cell phones at work, ask for an exception until your partner delivers, and promise to keep the phone on vibration mode.

Ask other support people to carry cell phones and keep them on as your partner's due date approaches.

What If You Have to Leave Town?

If you absolutely have to take an overnight trip during the five-week window when your partner's likely to go into labor, you need a backup plan.

Find a backup coach. This person should have some knowledge of birth and should be able to drop everything to help your partner. If you don't have a friend or family who fits these criteria, consider hiring a doula (page 23).

Enlist friends and family members. Have someone call the house every day to make sure your partner is feeling okay. She might even like to have a friend or relative stay with her.

Get to know your neighbors. In case your backup coach can't get to your partner in time, find out if one of your neighbors can drive her to the hospital if needed. (No matter what, your partner shouldn't drive herself to the hospital in labor. If no one is available and she has to get to the hospital fast, she should call for an ambulance.)

Talk to your boss. Find out whether you'll be able to leave at a moment's notice if your partner goes into labor, or whether you'll have to stay until the end of the day or even the end of the conference.

Figure out how you can get home fast. Program numbers for the airport, rental-car company, and train station on your cell phone, or keep the numbers close by. This way you'll be able to book a trip home quickly if your partner goes into labor while you're gone.

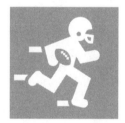

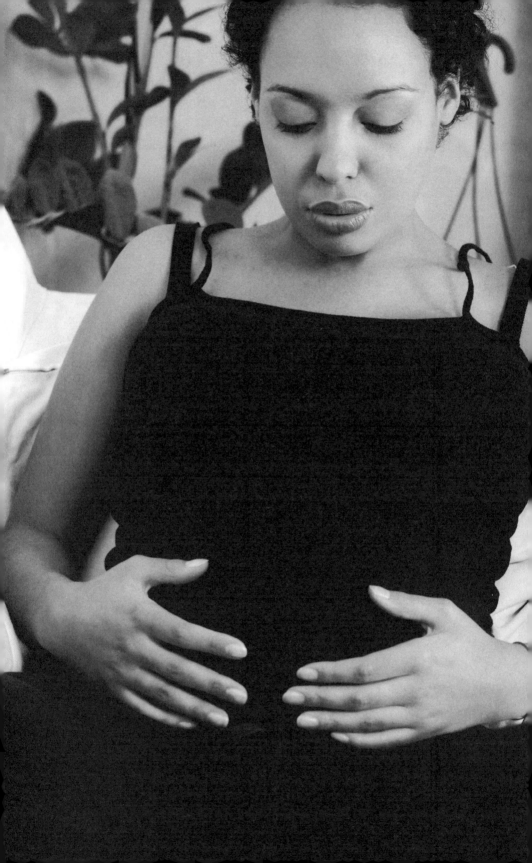

Chapter 3
"DOES IT HURT YET?"
and Other Things Not to Ask in Early Labor

 ou've done all the prep work for the birth. The bags are packed and you know who's going to be at the birth. You've taken your classes and you know the things that might happen before she goes into labor. In fact, you may have seen some of these things—has she shown you her mucus plug or some bloody show yet (see below)?

How Will You Know It's the Big Day?

Unfortunately, you may not. Some women go into labor suddenly, and others begin to ease into it weeks before the birth. But there are some things your partner may do that will let you know the baby is coming soon.

She may get cranky. Many women are cranky for a few weeks before labor begins, probably because of a combination of factors—hormonal changes, the discomfort of the last few weeks of pregnancy, and maybe even anxiety about the birth and becoming a mom. But if your partner suddenly begins snapping or cursing, she may be going into labor. If she bites off your head, try not to take it personally.

She may get depressed. She may say she hates her ankles, she hates her big belly, and this baby's never coming out. She may think her world is a big, dark pit of despair. If this is a new thing, maybe she's going into labor. Try to comfort her, or just let her wallow.

She may lose her mucus plug. This is a clump of mucus that helps seal the cervix. As the cervix starts to soften and open, the plug falls out. Your partner may lose her mucus plug all at once in the toilet or gradually over a day or two. She may even lose it several times, because it can recharge. You may hope she'll keep this matter to herself, and she may. But if she asks, "Honey, do you think this is my mucus plug?" just look for a big clump of mucus.

She may have "bloody show." This is mucus from the cervix again, but blood-tinged, because the capillaries in the cervix are popping. Especially for first-timers, bloody show is a good sign—an indication that things are getting going. A lot of blood, however, is an emergency—a signal to call the doctor or midwife immediately.

She may be cleaning the house. You come home from work to find that your partner is scrubbing the baseboards with a toothbrush, bleaching the fridge, or frantically pulling weeds. Or she hands you a honey-do list that's five pages long. Probably she's experiencing a nesting urge. Try to get her to take it easy. You don't want her to clean all day, then go to bed exhausted and desperate for a good night's sleep, because she'll probably go into labor that night.

She may have a lot of irregular contractions. Often labor begins with an increase in prelabor or Braxton-Hicks contractions (see page 163). In some women, these feel achy, like mild menstrual cramps. Over time, the contractions get stronger and more regular, until a woman finds herself in active labor. Prelabor contractions generally aren't painful (at least not as painful as the contractions of active labor) and should be manageable with comfort techniques or distractions.

She seems to have a mild case of stomach flu. If your partner is nauseated, vomiting, or experiencing some diarrhea, she may think she has food poisoning. It's more likely that her body is cleaning itself out, since the digestive system mostly shuts down during labor. Offer her foods that are easy on the stomach—like soup, rice, dry toast, and applesauce—to keep her energy up for the big day.

What If Prelabor Lasts for Weeks?

You've gotten that phone call from your partner saying she's in labor—five times now. Every time she thinks this is the real thing, her contractions fizzle out a few hours later. You've had so many practice runs to the hospital that the car could get there by itself. Both of you are getting frustrated, and you're wondering if this baby is ever going to come out. What do you do?

Talk to her doctor or midwife. Find out when you're supposed to go to the hospital, and don't jump the gun. You'll probably be told to go when the contractions are coming regularly between three and six minutes apart, when they each last sixty seconds, and when they have been this way for an hour or two. If you go in too early, the nurses will probably send you home, and no one likes that. If they don't send you home, your partner may end up getting Pitocin to augment her contractions, and that will increase the likelihood that she'll need an epidural. It's particularly important not to head in too early if your partner wants to go unmedicated.

Go for a walk. Walking may help get this show on the road. If nothing else, it will pass the time. But don't let your partner get exhausted; that would make her labor harder. Moderation is the key.

Have sex. As long as your partner's waters haven't broken, you should feel free to have sex. A massage may help get her in the mood. This may be the last time for a while, so enjoy it.

Encourage her to relax. Relaxation may make the contractions go away for a while so both of you can get some rest. When you wake up, they may escalate into true labor contractions. Pamper your partner with massage and her favorite movie or music while making sure you don't get too tired.

Rest. If you wear yourself out before labor begins, you won't be much help to your partner. Labor is a marathon, not a sprint.

Wait for the frown. At some point your partner will probably frown and say that her contractions feel different now. Most likely, these are the real deal. Instead of petering out, they'll get stronger, longer, and closer together.

Enjoy this time. Although you've been waiting months for the birth, you may later wish you'd had a few more days without the baby. Enjoy watching a movie all the way through, having a complete conversation with your partner, and sleeping straight through the night—because the days of no interruptions are almost gone.

When prelabor really hurts If your partner has been having strong contractions without a break for hours or days, but her cervix isn't changing, she may be experiencing prodomal labor. See page 101 for more information.

How and Why Do You Time Contractions?

You time contractions to find out if they're getting longer and closer together, so you'll know when to call the doctor or midwife and when to head to the hospital. Most birthing facilities don't want to hear from a laboring woman or her partner until the contractions follow the 4-1-1 rule (see page 49).

The 4-1-1 rule If your partner is a first-timer, the doctor or midwife will probably want to her to contact the hospital or them when her contractions are about four minutes apart, when they last a full minute each, and when they have been this way for an hour. This is called the 4-1-1 rule. If your partner has already had a baby or two, her doctor or midwife will probably want to see her earlier, when her contractions are, say, six to seven minutes apart. Check with the doctor or midwife so you know exactly when to call and when to go to the hospital.

Measure the frequency of contractions by timing from the start of one to the start of the next. Also time the length of a contraction. For example, let's say a contraction starts at 1:05 and lasts until 1:06. The next contraction starts at 1:08. In this case, the contraction lasted one minute and the contractions are three minutes apart, as you can see in the illustration.

Contractions are lasting 1 minute and are 3 minutes apart.

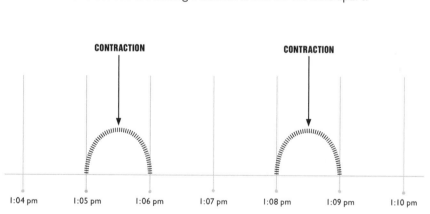

| CONTRACTION | | CONTRACTION |

| 1:04 pm | 1:05 pm | 1:06 pm | 1:07 pm | 1:08 pm | 1:09 pm | 1:10 pm |

Most men do a great job timing contractions, but some of them drive their partners crazy by timing every single one. Don't start timing until your partner tells you that her contractions are becoming longer, stronger, and closer together. Then check the pattern by timing every second or third one.

And don't take the term *coach* too literally by using a stopwatch; the clicking would annoy her. Any clock or wristwatch with a second hand will work fine. It doesn't matter if you're not measuring to the exact second.

Don't make it your one and only goal to time contractions. Your partner needs you for other things, like packing the car, blowing up the birthing ball (see page 163), getting her something to drink, playing a game with her, or turning on the shower.

Once you get to the birthing facility, you probably won't need to time contractions anymore. The staff will time them as needed with a fetal monitor (see page 83).

What Does Labor Feel Like?

Some people say that the closest men can come to experiencing labor pain is passing a kidney stone. In fact, some women who pass kidney stones find them much more painful than labor. In addition, the pain of kidney stones can last for days or weeks. (Unlike labor, of course, kidney stones don't cause hormonal upset. No one has ever had post-kidney-stone depression.)

Many women say that early labor contractions feel like menstrual cramps. In fact, menstrual cramps *are* light uterine contractions. You don't know what menstrual cramps feel like, of course, so this doesn't help you much. To give you a better idea, menstrual cramps are low, achy pains in the lower belly and sometimes the lower back. Some women say they're like intestinal cramps, though others disagree. Menstrual cramps don't bother some women at all, but they make others very uncomfortable every month.

Labor is like that, too—the intensity of the pain varies a lot. Some women experience excruciating pain from the beginning, but others feel virtually no pain (1 percent of the population, in fact—the odds are better than those of winning the lottery!). This is part of the reason you'll hear such varying reports about what labor feels like. Some people think it's the worst pain ever. Others say it hurts, but it's manageable.

The nice thing is that labor pain comes and goes. Unless your partner has back labor (see page 98), she'll have breaks between contractions when she won't feel any pain. There will probably be more break time than contraction time. In addition, contractions build and then let up. The peak of the contraction—the most painful part—lasts no longer than thirty seconds.

How Can You Help Your Partner Handle the Pain?

For 99 percent of women, giving birth hurts. This is true even for those who get an epidural as soon as possible. Your partner will probably undergo many contractions before she will be admitted to the hospital, and after that she may have to wait several hours before she can have an epidural, if she wants one. It will be hard for you to see her in pain, but the good news is that you can help her. Here's how:

Remember that pain is part of the process. We don't really know why birth hurts, but some people say that any kind of pain guides us to comfort. For example, when you walk around on a sprained ankle, it hurts. Your body is telling you, "Hey, moron, get off your ankle and let it heal!" Labor pain drives women to get into positions that both decrease the pain and help the baby to come out. This is why lying down during labor (which goes against gravity) makes contractions hurt more. Your partner needs to move around and try out various upright positions, and you can help her do this.

Help her deal with the pain in other ways. The worst thing you can do is tell her you don't know what to do. Pull out your cheat sheet (see page 34) and review your comfort measures. When contractions get hard, you can breathe with her, suggest that she close her eyes, or help her find a focal point. You can ease her pain with music, cool compresses, massage, and the shower.

Focus on the break time, not the contractions. Unless your partner has back pain (see page 98), she'll have breaks between contractions when she should be feeling no pain whatsoever. You can help her relax and enjoy this pain-free time.

Remember that it's her pain, not yours. Many well-meaning coaches object when their partners want to go entirely unmedicated or postpone an epidural. You may hate to see your partner hurting, especially when relief is only an epidural away. But it's her choice whether and when to use pain meds. Think about how angry she would be after the birth if she felt that you had forced her to take drugs she didn't want.

Remember that she needs you to be strong. If you start panicking, she'll panic. You must be a rock she can lean on, a rock she can depend on no matter what happens. The stronger you are, the stronger she'll be. So try to hold off on any emotional outbursts.

How can she be in labor if her waters haven't broken? You've been watching too many movies. In Hollywood, everyone's labor starts with a big gush of fluid from the vagina. In reality, though, only 10 to 12 percent of labors start with the spontaneous rupture of the amniotic sac, or "membranes."

What Do We Do If Her Waters Break?

The bag of waters can break with a gush or a trickle. If only a trickle of liquid is coming out, your partner may wonder whether it's amniotic fluid or urine, especially if she has experienced urine leakage in late pregnancy. Here's what to do:

If she's confused, have her empty her bladder. If she's still leaking continuously or every time she moves, it's amniotic fluid, not urine.

Get a towel. She'll continue to leak fluid until the baby's head drops down and blocks the birth canal. Some women experience a small gush of fluid with every movement and every contraction. So have her sit on a towel or put a thick menstrual pad or even a diaper in her underpants.

Check the fluid. Is it colored? Does it have a funky smell? Clear fluid with a light bleach-like or sweet smell is normal. The staff at the hospital will also want to know what time the water broke.

Call the doctor or midwife. The provider will want to know when the waters broke and what the fluid looks and smells like. The provider will probably ask you to head into the birthing facility or the provider's office right away. Once the amniotic sac has ruptured, bacteria can get into the uterus and cause a nasty infection. To minimize the chance of infection, most providers want the baby out within twenty-four hours of the waters' breaking. If strong contractions don't begin within a few hours, the provider will likely recommend Pitocin to get things moving. If any signs of infection appear or your partner has tested positive for Group B strep (see page 170), antibiotics will be started immediately.

Remind your partner not to introduce bacteria into the vagina. She shouldn't insert a tampon or a menstrual cup to catch the fluid, and the two of you shouldn't have intercourse. In addition, she should check with her doctor or midwife before taking a bath, though studies show that baths are safe after the bag of waters breaks.

Keep calm. The breaking of the bag of waters can be dramatic, but it's normal. You don't need to worry about the baby; only the fluid around the head has come out. There is still plenty of fluid around the baby's body, and the placenta should continue to make more until after the baby is born.

What to Do During Early Labor at Home

You think this is the big day. You're staying home from work. Contractions are coming closer together, and your partner is working a little harder during them. You've called your doctor or midwife, but you've been told to stay at home until contractions are a little stronger and closer together still. Now what do you do?

Tidy up. Refrigerate any food that would rot on the kitchen counter. Take out the garbage. Make sure your house is clean enough that your partner won't feel compelled to tidy up before friends and relatives drop in to meet the new baby.

Keep her busy. The worst thing you could do is to stare at her, waiting for a contraction to time. You'd only encourage her to dwell on her contractions, which would make them feel worse. When you exercise on a stationary bike, treadmill, or stair machine, do you watch television, read, or do mental exercises to pass the time? Distraction helps in early labor, too. Following is a list of things you can do to keep her mind off the contractions. (If you leave the house, remember to bring your bags with you, just in case.)

— See a movie.

— Go to the mall (but don't let her buy shoes—they won't fit after the birth).

— Go to a baby store to get into the parenting mood.

— Go for a walk.

— Have a picnic in the park.

— Go for a drive.

— Take a nap.

— Start a TV-show marathon—find out how *Lost* started or finally start watching *Mad Men*, *Game of Thrones*, or those other TV shows everyone's telling you to try!

— Have sex (she may be more interested than you'd think; see page 40).

— Play card, board, or video games together.

— Invite her mom, her sister, her best friend, or a neighbor over.

— Suggest that she call a friend or relative. If you like, have a three-way conversation by speaker phone.

— Give her a massage.

— Suggest one of her favorite pastimes—reading, hanging out on Facebook, sewing, scrapbooking, cooking, or whatever. Join in, if it's something the two of you like doing together.

Listen to her. In early labor, many women are excited, a little nervous, and very chatty.

Call your support people. Let them know they should be prepared to head to the birthing facility soon.

Feed her. Offer your partner a snack or light meal, but make sure it's easy to digest. Forget the pizza or McDonald's run; many women throw up in active labor. Your partner needs the sort of food you'd eat while recovering from the stomach flu. Warm up some soup, grill a cheese sandwich, or just give her some applesauce to keep her energy up. To prevent dehydration, also make sure she drinks plenty of liquids—water, juice, tea, or broth.

Feed yourself. This may be the last time you have a meal until after the baby's here. Share your partner's snack, or have something more filling—eggs, yogurt with fruit, or a sandwich. Avoid greasy foods or any food that might cause heartburn, gas, or bad breath. You don't need any such troubles while you're trying to help your partner with contractions.

Do any last-minute tasks. Imagine you're going to a cabin in the woods where no one will be able to find you. Let your boss know you may not be coming in tomorrow and put any scheduled meetings on hold. Make sure the bags are packed, the car has gas, and there will be food in the fridge when you get home from the hospital. Check your e-mail and update your voice mail. Don't forget to change into comfy clothes before you leave for the hospital.

Don't use that cheat sheet yet! This is a good time to help your partner get into a comfortable position—one that makes the contractions less bothersome—and to distract her however you can. This is also a good time to review breathing and massage techniques. But this is a bad time to try everything on the cheat sheet. If you massage your partner by candlelight while she lies in a warm bath before the contractions are truly making her uncomfortable, you run the risk that these things won't work when she really, really needs them. It's like turning your windshield wipers on high when it's only sprinkling. When it starts pouring, you get frustrated because you can't make the wipers move faster.

What to Do During Early Labor at the Hospital

Most women go to the hospital when they're in active labor. But some head in earlier, because they are considered "high risk" for some reason or because they're having labor induced (see page 166). If your partner is in one of these categories, the two of you will go through early labor— the longest part—in a place that may not be very comfortable or homey. What should you do?

Find a way to keep you both busy. There may be down time while you're waiting for contractions to get going. Play a game together, or watch a movie.

Have someone show you how to use the electronics. Ask the nurse to show you how to page her and how to work the CD player, the mp3 player dock, the TV, the DVD player, the phone, and any other nonmedical electronic equipment in the room. This way you won't fool around with the machinery and accidentally change some settings before realizing you don't know what you're doing and need the nurse or the janitor to fix everything.

Feel free to explore the room. If a cupboard isn't locked, peek inside. If you see towels, sheets, blankets, and washcloths, grab them—they're for your partner's use, and leaving them untouched won't get you a discount on the hospital bill. If you're not sure what something is, especially if it looks medical, don't touch it. You might set off an alarm or move supplies that the staff may need in an emergency.

Help her to get some rest. Make sure your partner is comfortable, and then lie down yourself (see page 86 for tips about sleeping in a hospital).

Ask the staff if your partner can eat. If contractions haven't really started, the nurses may let her have a meal. Otherwise they may allow "clear fluids"—juices, broths, Italian ices, flavored gelatin, and frozen juice bars. Many hospitals provide these things for laboring moms, so ask. Eating will give your partner the energy she'll need to get through her labor. Make sure you take time for a meal yourself.

Ask friends to bring you things you need or just stop by. Your friends can help you both pass the time until contractions get going. But let these people know that they may have to leave when things do get started, if that's what your partner wants.

Have patience. Especially if your partner's labor is being induced, getting contractions going and keeping them going can take a long time.

The Car Ride to the Hospital

In her doula days, after Theresa would join a couple at their home in early labor, she would follow them to the hospital in her own car. Theresa remembers one time when the dad was driving and the mom was in the back seat. Every time Mom had a contraction, her arm shot straight up to the ceiling of the car. And every time that happened the car swerved dramatically, making other cars swerve in response. Theresa almost called Dad on the cell to remind him to drive carefully, but she was worried this would distract him more. Luckily, they all made it to the hospital safely.

Imagine, now: Your partner's contractions are getting close together and strong. You're at home thinking it's time to get her to the hospital. But she needs you during every contraction—to rub her back, breathe with her, or talk to her. How are you going to drive and help her through the contractions at the same time?

Make her comfortable. If her waters haven't broken yet, put a towel on the back seat. Then help her in. Give her some pillows, a cool compress, and water to sip. Put on whatever music she wants to hear. If her back's killing her, give her an air-activated heating pad (see page 38). She also may need a bucket; many women throw up during labor.

Bring along a helper. It's very hard to drive safely when your partner is making worrisome noises and you're telling her to breathe, focus, concentrate, or relax. If possible, have someone else either do the driving or help your partner in the back seat.

Drive safely. If you have to do the driving, don't speed or run red lights; you don't want to arrive at the hospital by ambulance. If your partner starts groaning or making other noises, comfort her with words, but keep your eyes on the road and your hands on the wheel.

What if the baby starts coming on the way to the hospital? If you're worried you're not going to make it to the hospital before the baby comes, pull over and call 911. If you can see the baby's head, have the medic talk you through the delivery. Keep in mind, though, that the reason it makes the news whenever babies arrive in cars, taxis, and buses is because this doesn't happen very often. If you think you can't make it to your birthing facility but know there's another hospital close by, go there. You can work out payment later.

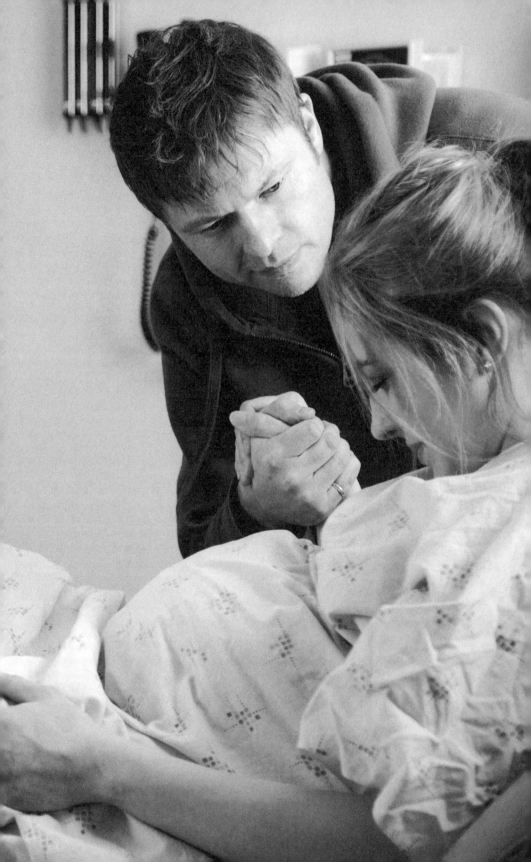

Chapter 4

YOU DIDN'T KNOW WHAT YOU WERE SIGNING UP FOR:
How to Help with Strong Contractions

ow things are getting intense. Your partner is officially in labor! You've confirmed it with her doctor or midwife, and you're at the birthing facility. Now you're in a strange room full of weird equipment and people you've never met who will see your partner's bits. There may also be support people whom you and your partner invited, so you might need to do some crowd control. Plus, your partner is starting to really need your help to get through contractions. Maybe she's starting to think about having an epidural, or maybe she remains committed to an unmedicated birth. Either way, she's starting to need some weird things.

How to Use the Room

For weeks now you and your partner have been practicing the labor positions you learned in your childbirth class, and you know which ones you want to use. But that position she loved in the recliner at home (not the one that led to your needing this book!) won't work so well here. You also don't know where the TV is (at one hospital we know of it's hidden in a cupboard) or where the extra towels are. What do you do?

Use your nurse. Page her if you can't get hot water in the shower, need extra pillows or towels, can't get the toilet to flush, or want an extra chair. Helping you is part of her job. As the nurse told us when Theresa was in labor, the squeaky wheel gets the grease.

Your nurse can be your best friend or your worst nightmare. If you don't like her or she's unhelpful, you can fire her. See page 70 for details.

Don't play with the baby warmer! See that bassinet-like thing hooked up to a lot of cords? That's where the baby goes if she needs a little extra help after birth. Don't touch it!

Learn how to unhook the fetal monitor. If your partner has to be hooked up to a fetal monitor (see page 83), you don't want to have to take it completely off each time she has to run to the bathroom. Ask the nurse to show you how to unhook the wires and how to hook them back in (it's very easy). Promise your nurse you'll get her approval before unhooking Mom.

Use the bed. You can raise the entire hospital bed so your partner can stand next to it, leaning her cheek against a birthing ball. Or you can raise just the head of the bed, so she can kneel and get a back massage while leaning forward against the raised mattress. You might even be able to make the hospital bed into a sort of chair (ask the nurse).

Use the bedside table. A hospital room always has a bedside table whose top fits over the bed. You can use this table to support your partner in various positions. You might raise the top and lock it into place for Mom to lean on as she gets a back rub. Just make sure you lock the wheels, or place a washcloth beneath them, so the table doesn't move.

Find the small stool. A six-inch-high stool may be a big help if your partner wants to slow-dance but you're an uncomfortable height for her. If she's short, the stool may also be useful for hopping in and out of bed or for sitting on while getting foot rubs. You might sit on the stool yourself while your partner is on the floor, in the shower, or in a birthing tub. If your room doesn't have a stool, ask for one. Every hospital should have a few.

Put down padding. Make everything around your partner as comfortable and soft as possible. If she wants to lie on the floor, lay blankets and sheets there (ask the nurse for extra blankets and sheets if you can't find them in your room). If your partner is sitting in a rocking chair, put a pillow behind her back. If she's leaning on a ball, put a pillow on it.

Your Comfort Is Important, Too!

One of the biggest mistakes dads make during labor is neglecting to take care of themselves. They think they shouldn't complain about a little neck, knee, or shoulder pain when their partners are in so much more pain. But if you're not comfortable, you can't be a good coach. One of the dads who tell their stories in Chapter 7 made this mistake. He got very sick during the birth and later felt that he hadn't helped much.

Use pillows to prevent back, shoulder, and knee pain. To prevent lower back pain, put a pillow behind your back when you sit in a chair. When you're resting, put your head on a pillow. When you're kneeling, keep a pillow under your knees or wear knee pads. This all seems like common sense, but in her classes Theresa sees dads ignoring their own comfort all the time. And she knows of an inexperienced doula (okay, okay, it was Theresa, during one of the first births she attended) who injured herself because she wouldn't use a pillow to make herself more comfortable.

Take medicine, if you need it. If your back, shoulder, or knees are seizing up, take an anti-inflammatory such as ibuprofen. Tylenol will also work. Avoid strong painkillers such as codeine or Vicodin, which could affect your coaching ability.

Ask another support person for a massage. One of the great things about additional support people is that they can take care of you. If you're hurting, ask for a shoulder or back massage. Theresa attended one birth that featured a chain massage: While the dad was massaging the mom's back, Theresa massaged his shoulders—and then a nurse started rubbing Theresa's shoulders!

Wear comfortable clothes. Remember the sweatpants and T-shirt you packed in your bag? If you're not wearing comfortable clothes now, change. If you're cold, put on your sweatshirt or jacket.

Sit on a chair or stool. Theresa has seen many dads squatting behind their partners or sitting directly on cold hard floors, and then shifting positions a few minutes later, while wincing and rubbing their knees and backs. Grab a chair or stool to sit on while supporting your partner.

Take a power nap. When you're not actively supporting your partner—for example, she's in the shower, she has told you to leave her alone, or she has fallen asleep after getting an epidural—sit or lie down. Close your eyes and nap (see page 86 for advice about sleeping in a hospital). Even five minutes of sleep will help energize you to keep supporting your partner.

Protect the Space

Theresa attended a birth during California's election of Arnold Schwarzenegger as governor. All the TVs were tuned to the election, and every staff person who came into the room commented on it. The laboring woman and her partner asked for the TV to be turned off so they could focus on the contractions, not on the election results. Still, every time a nurse came into the room she turned on the TV so she wouldn't miss anything. This sort of thing happens more often than you'd think.

A good birthing space is relatively quiet and dim. Voices should be low and music at a comfortable level; very few women want to give birth at a rave. If the TV is on, it should be set to your partner's favorite channel or show. This means no sporting events—even if it's the Super Bowl or the World Series—unless she likes them.

Here are other ways to protect the space:

Use the dimmer switch, or pull the blinds on the windows. If you can't reduce the amount of light in the room and it's bothering your partner, give her a dry washcloth or an eye mask to cover her eyes.

Put on music. Music can keep the noise and chaos of the hospital at bay. Play something the two of you have picked beforehand. Don't be surprised if your partner wants to change the music a lot during labor, and be prepared to help her do this. If she doesn't want music but doesn't want quiet either, recorded nature sounds or a white-noise machine should do. She could also use earplugs or headphones/earbuds if she wants.

Keep voices soft. Loud voices can break your partner's concentration. Remind your other support people to keep their voices soft by speaking in a soft voice yourself.

Use scents. If you've brought a pillow from home, it may have a comfortingly familiar smell. If your partner likes aromatherapy products and the hospital allows them, spritz some around the room, use a scented LED candle (a flickering, battery-operated lightbulb), or give your partner a bottle or cup containing a cotton ball soaked in an essential oil.

Crowd Control

Remember all those people you and your partner asked to be at the birth? They're all here, filling up the hospital room, asking a lot of questions, gossiping, and getting in the way. Now you have to figure out how to manage them.

Don't call people If you're concerned that friends and family members will show up uninvited if you or your partner calls to say she's in labor, then don't call until after the baby is born, or about to be born. If they complain, just say you were too busy to call any sooner.

Remember that Mom's in charge. Your partner may have thought she'd want fifteen people to witness the birth, but she may change her mind halfway through labor. You may have to play bouncer (see "How to Kick Someone Out," page 67). Or she may have thought she would want only you present, but suddenly she wants her mother and sister there, too. Be flexible, and read page 152 about a dad who wasn't sure he wanted his partner's mom and sister at the birth, but changed his mind once he saw how helpful they were.

Set ground rules. If you've talked with your partner about her desires for the birth, you know what to tell friends and family to do. Loud voices and the television on may or may not be okay. Some women want people around chatting and having fun, but others want everyone to be quiet. Review the discussion of extroverts and introverts on page 4 if you're confused.

Control odors. Smelly foods like coffee or French fries can make laboring moms nauseated or hungry. Many hospitals don't allow women to eat in labor. If your partner smells those fantastic French fries, gets hungry, and can't eat, she's going to get cranky. At you. People who want to eat should leave the room. Also, make sure nobody bothers your partner with their perfume, aftershave, or even body odor.

Don't let the labor room turn into a living room. Sometimes support people at a birth get bored and look for ways to entertain themselves. Don't let anyone put on their favorite music or turn on the football game and cheer for their favorite team. And make sure your support people watch what they say among themselves. Most important, put a quick stop to any horror stories about births or hospitals. Just catching someone's eye and shaking your head may do the trick. Your partner will thank you later.

Remember that you're number 2. No one other than your partner can kick you out of the room. Her mother, sister, or best friend shouldn't ask you to leave. In fact, these other people should be taking care of you. They should be making sure you're getting something to eat, taking restroom breaks, and getting a longer break occasionally if you need it. As the father of the baby, you have rights.

How to kick someone out Before the birth, warn the other support people that your partner might want them to leave at some point. Have your partner choose a code word. When she uses this word (*ice cream*, oddly enough, is a popular choice), she's saying, "Get these people the heck out!" Then, be the bad guy. Kick people out, and keep them out. Tell them you'll give them an update as soon as something changes. Enlist the nurse's help, if necessary.

Dealing with the Hospital Staff

Once you get to the hospital, you and your partner aren't alone anymore. Now you have to deal with strangers, medical experts with jobs to do. They are there to help you and your partner, but their primary job is the medical side of birth and the health of your partner and the baby. These people can make a huge difference in how smoothly the birth goes. Here's how to deal with them:

Introduce yourself. Shake hands with each person who walks into the labor room, or at least give a nod. If possible, tell everyone your name and your partner's name, and ask for their names. This seems simple, but the intensity of labor can make it hard to remember to be courteous.

Use their names. Call the nurses and doctors by name, and make eye contact when you speak with them. If you're bad at remembering names, you're in luck: They will be wearing name badges.

Be nice. No matter what's going on with the labor or how the staff is treating you, smile as much as possible, and say "please" and "thank you" when asking for things. If the nurses like you and think you're polite, you're more likely to get what you want.

Make jokes. Jokes make us seem more human and less like random strangers. Even if your jokes are bad, try dropping a few to see if you can get some smiles out of the staff. At worst, you'll keep your partner's mind off the contractions while she's telling you to knock it off.

Get to know the staff. If you have down time (which usually happens when a woman gets an epidural), ask the staff about themselves. Find out if they have kids, pets, or interesting hobbies. If they comment on the music you're listening to, find out about their musical interests. Ask what they think of popular movies or TV shows. This sort of small talk makes you and your partner seem more personable, so you're more likely to get extra help. But keep the conversation light; steer away from discussions of religion, politics, or birthing and parenting philosophies.

Don't be afraid to ask for help. It does no good to go to the hospital prepared to "do battle" for the kind of birth you and your partner want. Instead, let the nurse know your goals by presenting your birth plan. Then ask for her help. If your partner wants to go unmedicated, let the nurse know you would love any tips she could offer. If your partner wants to breastfeed immediately after birth, tell your nurse you'll need help with that. Your nurse is a fountain of knowledge, and if you ask she'll be willing to share that knowledge with you.

Ask for clarification. If you don't understand what a staff member is trying to tell you, say so. The staff deal with birth daily; you'll probably do it no more than a few times in your entire life. In addition, chances are you're feeling emotional and tired, and you may be hungry, too. Your partner is feeling the same things while dealing with contractions. This can make comprehending technical terms a lot harder. You need to understand what's going on so you can explain it to your partner, if need be. Read "Birth Jargon Explained," pages 162 to 171, to familiarize yourself with terms the staff may use.

Stop the staff from talking to your partner during contractions. She won't be able to focus on what they're saying. But, again, be polite.

Ask the staff to wait outside while you and your partner make decisions. If someone comes into the room to suggest an intervention, such as breaking the bag of waters, and you and your partner want to discuss the intervention before agreeing to it, ask the staff nicely to leave. This way you'll feel less pressure as you decide. If the staff won't leave, a doula we know suggests that you say you'd like some privacy to pray for guidance.

Vent out of earshot. If you don't like your nurse or you're frustrated about what's going on, don't complain within the hearing range of the staff. You might offend them, and then they won't be as helpful to you and your partner.

If necessary, ask for a new nurse. If you and your partner don't like the nurse or you think her birthing philosophy conflicts with yours (for example, your partner wants to go unmedicated but the nurse is pushing for an epidural), feel free to ask for a new nurse. Just go out to the nurses' station and ask to talk to the charge nurse or the nurse-manager. Then ask this person to assign someone else to your partner. Don't worry about offending the rejected nurse; chances are the bad feelings are mutual and your nurse will be happy to get a different patient.

Bribing the Hospital Staff

This is an old doula trick: A bribe makes the nurses a little friendlier and a little more willing to help you and your partner realize your plans for the birth. When you go to a trade show, each company hands out candies, pencils, or the like in the hope that you'll favor their business. This is just what you're trying to do with the nurses. Here are some suggestions:

Bring food. Buy some cookies or doughnuts on the way to the hospital, or bake some brownies during early labor at home. In case some of the nurses are watching their diets, you might instead choose a tray of raw vegetables, fruit, nuts, cheese, or pieces of dark chocolate.

Choose small inedible gifts. Before labor begins, check out the bins of notepads, mini-massagers, and picture frames at a dollar store. Get a variety of things, and let each nurse choose one.

Bring plenty of the bribes you choose. Your primary nurse may have to attend another patient or go to lunch, or her shift may end, and so you'll have a new nurse needing a bribe. Or your nurse may be accompanied by a student who also wants a goody. A technician may drop in, if only because word is getting around. Make sure you have at least five bribes on hand.

Protecting Your Partner's Modesty

One of the more important things a guy can do for a shy woman is to protect her modesty. Childbirth is inherently an immodest experience. The staff will do vaginal exams to check how far your partner's cervix has opened, and they'll probably massage her perineum, the skin between her anus and vagina, to decrease the likelihood of a tear occurring while she's pushing out the baby. When that baby is coming out, all their attention will be on your partner's privates. Then the nurses will probably bare Mom's chest so they can place the baby between her breasts (this is called skin-to-skin contact; see page 124). Now, some women don't care in the least about who sees what, so make sure you ask her ahead of time how modest she thinks she's going to be in labor. If your partner doesn't care about modesty in labor, feel free to skip this section (2 minutes saved!).

If the idea of having her body exposed to strangers scares your partner, there are some things you can do to help:

Use a sheet. Insist that the nurse cover your partner's privates with a sheet when doing vaginal exams. The nurse can simply lift the sheet from the bottom to insert her fingers. She doesn't even need to look much; the exam is based on feel rather than sight. Afterward, she may leave the sheet up, exposing your partner's privates. Ask the nurse to drop the sheet, or just drop it yourself.

Although your partner is expected to hold the baby against her bare skin after the birth, they can both be covered with a sheet. The sheet will help keep the baby warm, anyway.

Ask extra people to leave during procedures that require exposure. Your partner may be exposed not only during vaginal exams and while pushing the baby out. If her doctor breaks her bag of waters (see page 110) or inserts an electrode for internal fetal monitoring (see page 83), again her privates are going to be exposed. If she gets an epidural, the anesthesiologist will open her gown in the back. People in the room may see the top of her butt, and her hospital gown may slip down in front, exposing her breasts. During any of these procedures, staff members may make personal comments that your partner wouldn't want others to hear. For example, during a vaginal exam Theresa once heard a nurse say she could feel the poop in the mother's colon. So you may want to ask friends and family members to leave the room when it's time for any such procedure.

Watch that hospital gown. Hospital gowns come in different types, but they all gap in strange ways. Some open in the back to show off the butt; others open at the side to display the legs and hips. Some have snaps that come undone easily. As your partner moves around the room or turns in the bed, she may expose a breast, her butt, or even her privates. Help her stay covered with sheets or even pillows.

Suggest that your partner leave her bra on through labor. She may be more comfortable with a bra, anyway, if her breasts are large. It's best if she chooses a nursing bra (if she prefers sports bras, she can get one with cup flaps) or a bra that unhooks in the front, so she can easily make her breasts accessible to the baby after birth.

Suggest that she leave on her underpants, too. Wearing underpants and a menstrual pad may help your partner feel better if her waters have broken and fluid is leaking down her legs, although the nurse will ask her to remove the pants and pad periodically for vaginal checks. The hospital can probably even provide disposable underpants (one size fits all—sexy!).

Protect her modesty in the tub or shower. Some laboring women wear a bra or the top of a two-piece bathing suit in the shower or tub. Theresa knows of one woman who labored in a tub wearing the top of a tankini suit along with a skirt that covered her privates. The woman left off the suit bottom, but the skirt kept her privates covered. A towel can also provide covering when support or staff people come in to talk, so keep one handy if your partner's wearing nothing else.

Ask for privacy for the first breastfeeding. Again, this is a time when a modest mom may not want a lot of people in the room.

Are hospital gowns required? Not necessarily, though some hospitals and some doctors insist on them. (At one of the hospitals where Theresa works, a certain anesthesiologist refuses to give an epidural unless the woman is wearing a hospital gown.) However, if your partner thinks she'll be more comfortable laboring in a long T-shirt, a tank top and skirt, or a skirt and a bra, you can ask if the hospital will let her wear her own clothes. (Make sure she knows there's a chance that her clothes will get stained.)

Fun with Focal Points

When a woman is in labor, a focal point is something that she stares at during contractions to help her deal with the pain. Staring at the focal point may help her focus on her breathing or just give her something else to think about—like a favorite vacation place, if the focal point is a photo of that place. You may already use focal points all the time without realizing it. During a meeting at work, have you ever found yourself staring at a particular person or at an object on the table while you're thinking? When watching a sporting event, have you ever stared at a player or something on the field or court while thinking of something else entirely? In either case, the person or thing you've stared at is a focal point. A focal point in labor can be anything in the room. And the focal point is something you and your partner both can have some fun with.

If your partner thinks she might want to use a picture as a focal point, hopefully you'll have brought one along. But she may also want to stare at your face. This may feel awkward to you, but your face may become her anchor to get her through the contractions. Do your best to avoid making faces or otherwise trying to be funny unless this seems to help her deal with the contractions. Think calm and serene.

Some women choose a random object in the room to stare at—a bit of fuzz on the bed, a cellophane wrapper on the floor, a stain on the ceiling, or a sign on the wall. If this happens, notice what your partner's looking at, and don't block her view. She might hit you to make you move—ouch!

A student in one of Theresa's childbirth classes used a scrap of paper on the floor as her focal point. Unaware of what she was looking at, her husband stepped on the paper during a contraction. She "nearly ripped his kidney out" to get him to move, she said. When her epidural was administered, he put the bit of paper where she could see it. She later took the paper home from the hospital and put it in her baby book. She couldn't have gotten through labor without it, she said.

A few women like to stare at a clock or at the fetal monitor during contractions; this reminds them that contractions do end. For most women, though, staring at a clock or monitor makes a contraction feel a lot longer. It's like staring at the readout on a treadmill or exercise bike. The focal point is supposed to get your partner's mind off the contraction, not keep it there. To help keep your partner from staring at the clock and monitor, avoid staring at them yourself.

Keep the focal point in view If your partner's focal point is movable, put it where she can see it while she's getting an epidural started, an intravenous (IV) line placed, her waters broken (see page 110), or an electrode inserted for internal fetal monitoring (see page 83).

Using Ice Chips

Ask guys what they think they'll do to help their partners during labor, and most will say, "Find the ice machine and give her ice chips." Ice chips are readily available in most hospitals. They can keep a woman hydrated, and they help with the dry mouth that comes from using breathing techniques. Sucking or chewing on ice chips is also a great distraction. The more distracted your partner is, the less pain she'll feel.

Here are a few tips about using ice chips:

Know where and how to get them. Ask your nurse where the ice chips are and what container you should put them in. In some hospitals, the nurse will get them for you, in others you have to get them. In an ideal world, you've taken a tour ahead of time and asked someone so you already know how to get the ice chips.

Offer only a few at a time. Don't hand your partner a cup full of ice chips; she might choke on them or spit them all over you. Instead, offer just a few on a spoon or in a cup.

Be prepared for her to spit them out. Even if you've given her only one or two ice chips, your partner may suck them avidly between contractions but then spit them out when a contraction comes. Give her a container to spit into, or just let her spit the ice onto her gown. Be sure to offer more ice chips once the contraction is over.

Make them taste better. If the hospital and care provider allow, pour a little flavored syrup on the ice chips as an extra treat. (If your partner has gestational diabetes, she can't have sugar syrup.)

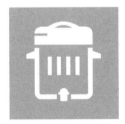 *Alternatives to ice chips* Your partner may prefer flavored gelatin or frozen juice bars over ice. If the hospital doesn't provide these (ask!), you can bring them from home. Gelatin and juice bars provide a little sugar that can help your partner get through the labor and birth. Always check with the doctor or midwife, though, before offering them.

Feeding Yourself

Don't forget to take time to eat some of those snacks you brought along in your bag. Eating may keep you from fainting, and it will also boost your energy for coaching and enjoying the bonding experience just after the baby is born. Here are some tips about eating during labor:

Grab one bite at a time. You may not have time for more. This is why we recommend energy bars; you can pull one from your pocket, take a bite, and then put the rest back in your pocket. (See page 36 for a discussion about the foods to put into your birthing bag.)

Get both a carb and a protein boost. Sugars and starches give you bursts of energy, but they can also leave you feeling a little shaky later on. Protein-rich foods like meat provide energy over the long term but won't perk you up right away. When you can take several minutes to eat, choose something with both protein and carbohydrates, such as dairy products, a sandwich, or, again, an energy bar.

Watch the smells. Do not eat pizza, French fries, eggs, bacon, sandwiches with onions, or other stinky foods in the labor room. Even the smell of coffee can make a laboring woman vomit. After you eat, be sure to grab a breath mint or rinse your mouth with water.

Drink plenty of fluids. Getting dehydrated would make you feel tired, and a tired coach is an ineffective coach. Water is the best choice for keeping hydrated, but a drink like Gatorade will keep your energy up as well. Soda with caffeine is good, too (says this pair of caffeine addicts), but if you haven't eaten for hours it can upset your stomach and make you jittery. Be especially careful of energy drinks like Red Bull, Rockstar, and Jolt, as they can make you very jittery if you're not used to them.

Why women aren't allowed to eat during labor
Many hospitals continue to forbid eating during labor. One hospital Theresa knows even frowns on giving ice chips! The reasoning, based on old practices and liability concerns, goes like this: *If* Mom gets a c-section and *if* she needs general anesthesia (if she's knocked out for the surgery, that is), and *if* there is food in her stomach, she *might* vomit and *might* inhale some of the vomit (although this is very unlikely if the doctors use a stomach tube, which they should) and so *might* get sick. Notice all those *ifs* and *mights*? The good news is that most women don't want to eat much during labor, so a sip of Gatorade, a smoothie, or broth may be all your partner wants. Be sure to talk to the doctor or midwife about the hospital's policy concerning food in labor.

Taking Breaks

Many wonderful men will not leave their partners' sides during labor. Although this is sweet and admirable, it's also stupid. You need to take breaks, especially if labor is long, for your physical and mental health. Now, we're not talking about thirty-minute breaks. We're talking about taking five minutes to eat, go to the bathroom, or walk the hall. Here are some tips:

Let your partner know you're leaving. Do not suddenly disappear. Between contractions, tell your partner you're going to take a break after the next contraction is done. Support her during the next contraction, and then go. During early and active labor her contractions will probably be three to ten minutes apart, so you will have plenty of time to pee or grab a quick bite before the next contraction starts.

Don't wait too long before taking a break. During transition (see page 171), there will be less time between contractions, and the contractions will be much more intense. It will be too late at this point to take a break; your partner will probably need your constant help. And you definitely shouldn't leave when it comes time for your partner to push, unless you're planning to be out of the room when the baby emerges.

Get help before taking a longer break. If for some reason you need to be away for more than a few minutes, or if you need a bathroom break when the contractions are very close together, find someone else to help your partner. If you don't have another support person, page the nurse.

Keeping Mom Cool

A big priority for you should be keeping your partner cool. The hard work of labor, combined with the effect of hormones, makes most laboring women boiling hot (though there are exceptions—see the sidebar for advice about dealing with a cold mom). Besides offering ice chips, there are other, often overlooked ways of keeping a woman cool.

Adjust the room temperature. The hospital may let you keep the room thermostat turned down low through most of labor. When it comes time to push, though, the staff will turn up the heat so the room will be warm for the baby.

Fan your partner. Take out your battery-operated fan and get it going. If you haven't brought a fan, fan your partner with a piece of paper folded up accordion-style.

Give her cold water to drink. Not only will water keep her cool, it will also prevent dehydration, which would be bad for the baby and would make your partner feel crappy.

What if she's cold? Some women shiver during labor, in response to either hormones or epidural medication. If your partner is cold, ask for some warmed blankets (hospitals keep blankets warm for the babies). Wrap her up; turn up the room temperature, if possible; and hug her.

Apply cool compresses. Put several washcloths in a basin of water with a little ice. When you want to apply one, squeeze it until it's just damp, not dripping. Lay it on your partner's chest, the back of her neck, her wrist, or her forehead (Theresa used to place cool compresses under the arms, too, until several women told her they didn't like wet armpits). Change the compresses after every third or fourth contraction. If the contractions are so close together that you don't have time to change compresses, just flip them over.

Keeping your partner cool in the shower Women who get into the shower to ease the pain of contractions usually feel much better right away. After a few minutes, though, they usually want out; they're too hot. Warm water may be perfect on the belly or back, but it may make the rest of a laboring body uncomfortably hot. You can encourage your partner to stay in the shower longer by giving her cold water to drink, ice chips to suck, or cool compresses for her neck or forehead.

Breathing Techniques

Although both moms and their coaches often overlook it, controlled breathing is one of the easiest and most effective ways to cope with labor. If breathing techniques are going to help your partner during contractions, however, she may need your help.

Since you may have already learned about breathing techniques in childbirth class, on the Internet, or through other books, we'll just review the basic techniques.

Cleansing breath. A deep breath or a deep sigh at the beginning or end of a contraction gives extra oxygen to the mom and the baby. More oxygen means less pain for your partner. A cleansing breath also lets you know when a contraction is beginning or ending. If your partner is still tense at the end of a contraction, have her take a cleansing breath or two to release the tension.

Slow-paced breathing. The many different names for this technique include yoga breathing and abdominal breathing. Women do slow-paced breathing in different ways. Typically, moms breathe in through their noses and out through their mouths. Some women are more comfortable breathing both in and out through their noses or through their mouths, and others will change from mouth to nose or nose to mouth during a contraction. Some moms focus on breathing all the way down into their abdomens, while others simply focus on inhaling and exhaling. Any variation is fine. The only thing for your partner to remember is to focus on her breathing.

Patterned breathing. This is the hee-hee-hee-blow technique. Your partner takes three short in-and-out breaths followed by one long exhalation, while you count her breaths on your fingers. She will need someone to demonstrate the technique so she doesn't hyperventilate, and the two of you will need to practice together to figure out a good rhythm. The power in this pattern is in its distracting difficulty; a person has to concentrate hard to do it properly. Many women find that they dislike using this technique in labor, but we advise practicing it anyway in case it may help.

Tips for Helping with Breathing Techniques

It's not enough to know the breathing techniques; you also need some guidelines for using them.

Don't tell your partner how to breathe. A laboring mom needs to listen to her body, not just to relieve her pain but also to get enough oxygen to her baby. If you correct your partner ("No! Breathe like this!"), you're going to make her angry, and she may panic.

If she starts to panic, help her. If your partner starts yelling, screaming, making higher-pitched noises, or flailing around, simply remind her to focus on her breathing. This will help her control her panic. See page 95 for more advice about dealing with a panicking mom.

If she gets noisy, let her. Many women like making noises during contractions. Some pray, some grunt or moan (as they might during sex), and some say the same words over and over. Don't interfere if your partner does any of these things, and try to avoid laughing unless you think this will help her relax.

Copy her breathing—maybe. Breathing with your partner during contractions may help her stay focused. Or it may annoy her. Follow your instincts about trying this. Once you start, check with her periodically to make sure you're not annoying her.

Get in her face—maybe. Your partner may like you to keep your face close to hers while you copy her breathing pattern, or she may not. She may like it in early labor and then hate it later. Go with your instincts, check with your partner occasionally, and don't get mad if getting in her face seems to help for a while but then she swats you away or tells you to knock it off.

Follow her rhythm—maybe. Nodding your head, moving your hand up and down, or tapping your foot to the rhythm of her breathing may help your partner when labor get intense. Or it might annoy her. Don't take offense if it doesn't help.

Supporting Your Partner During Monitoring

The word monitoring, as applied to labor, means measuring the baby's heartbeat and the mother's contractions. Every woman, whether she's delivering in a hospital, at home, or in a birthing center, will undergo some sort of monitoring. Periodically checking the baby's heartbeat may help in predicting problems before they become emergencies. Measuring the timing or strength of contractions, or both, helps in gauging the progress of labor.

Types of Monitors

There are several kinds of monitoring devices. At home births and in birth centers, midwives often use hand-held ultrasound stethoscopes, or Dopplers, to measure the baby's heartbeat. The fetal stethoscopes you see in old movies are hardly ever used anymore.

Hospitals rarely use hand-held monitors of any kind. The type of monitor they routinely use instead has sensors for both the baby's heartbeat and the mother's contractions (their timing, not their strength) in a belt or girdle that's strapped to the mom's abdomen. Wires connect the belt or girdle to a machine that continuously prints a strip of paper with graphs of both the baby's heartbeat and the contractions. This set of equipment is called an external monitor. The wires are several feet long, so during monitoring your partner can still stand, sit on a birthing ball or in a rocking chair, or get on her hands and knees.

An internal monitor is similar to an external one, except that the sensors are threaded through the birth canal. The contraction sensor, or intrauterine pressure catheter (IUPC), is placed next to the baby's head to monitor the strength as well as the timing of contractions. The fetal electrode, which monitors the baby's heartbeat, is poked slightly into the skin on the top of the baby's head. Care providers use internal monitors if they're having difficulty finding the baby's heartbeat, if the baby's heartbeat seems irregular, or if the uterus is contracting but the cervix isn't opening. Internal monitoring is used only when very accurate measurements of the contractions and the baby's heartbeat are needed. Although some providers allow laboring women with internal monitors to get out of bed, most do not. Unless her provider tells you otherwise, though, your partner can still sit up in bed, which will be much more comfortable during contractions than lying down.

In hospitals and some birth centers, the external or internal monitor is connected to a computer in the nurses' station, where the graphs are displayed on a video screen.

Intermittent Versus Continuous Monitoring

External monitoring is done intermittently—once each hour, for fifteen to twenty minutes at a stretch—if the mother is healthy, there are no special concerns about the baby, and the mom isn't on Pitocin, analgesics, or an epidural. If your partner doesn't meet these qualifications, she'll be monitored continuously. This will probably mean that she can't walk the halls or take a shower, though some hospitals have portable monitoring units, and sometimes they are waterproof.

Even with continuous external fetal monitoring, the hospital will probably let your partner get off the monitor to run to the bathroom as long as she promises to come back quickly. Unhooking the monitor is very easy, so have your nurse show you how to do it.

Internal monitoring is always continuous, however, and Mom is likely not getting disconnected for any reason. If she doesn't have a urinary catheter, she'll be offered a bed pan.

Don't stare at the monitor It may be interesting to watch graphical evidence of when contractions begin and end, and reassuring to see the pattern of the baby's heartbeat, but you shouldn't watch the monitor instead of helping your partner. She might feel you're ignoring her.

Supporting a Woman with an Epidural

Your partner just got her epidural, and it's working great. You may be thinking your job is done. But your partner still needs a good deal from you as she labors with the epidural. Here's how you can help:

Don't leave. Just because her pain is mostly gone doesn't mean she's not struggling emotionally. Unless she orders you to get out, stay in the room. If you need to make a phone call or grab something to eat, wait until she falls asleep or ask if the nurse can sit with her for a few minutes. Now is not the time to run home to shower, go car shopping (we know someone who did!), or go back to work.

Offer her sips of water, and keep her cool. Her body is still laboring, even if she can't feel it. She may still be hot and sweaty, and her mouth may get dry. Offer her cool compresses and small sips of water to keep her comfortable.

Let her rest. If labor has been long, she may want to sleep. Help her arrange the pillows and get into a comfortable position. Because she can't move her legs well, it may be hard for her to get her hips comfortable. Make the room as quiet as possible, and turn down the lights or offer her something to cover her eyes.

Help her change positions frequently. One of the biggest complaints about epidurals is that they cause back pain. For some women, though, back and hip pain immediately after birth may be caused by staying in the same position for too long. To prevent such pain, make sure your partner changes position about every thirty minutes. This will also help keep pain relief from the epidural consistent (some women get relief on only one side), and it may help the baby wiggle through the pelvis, so that labor may be shorter and your partner may be less likely to need Pitocin to keep contractions going.

Make sure she gets a urinary catheter. Women who get epidurals have difficulty urinating, because they are numb. If your partner gets an epidural, a urinary catheter will probably be inserted to keep her bladder empty. In this case, her urine will collect in a plastic bag hanging off the bed. Sometimes, though, a nurse gives a woman a bedpan instead of a catheter. Unless there's a medical reason that your partner can't have a catheter, ask for one. It's more comfortable for everyone.

Help her cope with any pain. About 15 percent of women who get epidurals don't get adequate pain relief. So, even with the epidural, your partner may appreciate massage or need help with breathing or focusing. (If the epidural truly isn't working, talk to the nurse and anesthesiologist, and see page 108 for tips.)

Help with pushing. Pushing with an epidural is usually harder than without; it's like walking on a leg that's gone numb, or talking after getting dental work done. You can help by encouraging her, holding her legs, helping her count, and keeping her cool with sips of water and compresses. For more advice on this topic, see page 115.

Sleeping at the Hospital

If your partner gets an epidural or the hospital lets you spend the night after your baby is born, you'll want to get some sleep. But where? Most hospitals don't let somebody curl up with the patient in a hospital bed— and hospital beds are too small for two people anyhow. Besides, if your partner is in labor with an epidural and you crawl in beside her, you might accidentally pull out important tubes and wires.

So look around the room. Is there a sleep couch or a chair that folds out into a bed (once you figure out how)? If not, you may have to get imaginative. Theresa remembers one dad who put two armchairs together, with the seats facing each other, and curled up on this little bench to sleep. She's seen dads sleep on window seats, tables, rocking chairs, and even the floor (she doesn't recommend the floor).

While it may help you to sleep if you use earbuds or earplugs, you shouldn't use them in this situation in case your partner needs help while you're sleeping.

Hospitals can be cold places, so page the nurse, if necessary, to ask for a pillow and blanket. If the hospital won't spare these for you, use the sweatshirt or jacket that you packed.

Get your feet up. It's easier to sleep in a chair if you can plant your feet on a wall or on another chair. But don't put them on your partner's bed or on any medical equipment.

Talking to Your Partner in Labor

When your partner is in labor, you can't talk to her as you normally would. She's uncomfortable, emotional, and hormonal. She does not understand you as easily, and she may have a shorter fuse. Knowing how to talk to her can prevent confusion and hurt feelings. Here are some tips:

Use clear and direct language. But don't piss her off by talking to her as you would to a child.

Wait until the contraction ends. During a contraction, she's focusing on getting through it; she can't concentrate on what you're saying. Don't say, "Honey, your mom just got here" or "Do you know where the cafeteria is?" or "How do you work the nurse's call button?" until after the contraction is over. Unless she tells you to shut up, though, it's okay to say *some* things during contractions—that she's doing a good job, that the contraction is almost over, that she should breathe through the pain, and so on.

Don't ask open-ended questions. Even between contractions, your partner won't be able to answer questions like "What do you want?" or "What do you want me to do?" Phrase your questions so she can answer yes or no: "Do you want to try the shower now?" "Do you want a hand massage?"

Take some initiative. Sometimes women in labor don't know what they want. If your partner asks what you think she should do, tell her. If your idea doesn't work, suggest something else for the next contraction. Don't shrug and tell her to do whatever feels good. She doesn't know what feels good to her at this point.

Explain things over and over. Laboring women often need multiple explanations or reminders. Don't get frustrated if your partner forgets something you've just told her.

Explain what the staff is trying to do or say. Your partner may not understand what doctors or nurses are trying to tell her. She may respond better to your familiar voice and diction. This is why you need to understand common obstetric procedures and terms (see "Birth Jargon Explained," pages 162 to 171).

Does she want a massage or not? Some women will suddenly slap their partners' hands away during massages. If your partner does this, it can mean either of two things. First, she may be associating your touch with pain. Keeping a hand on her between contractions may keep her from getting annoyed at your touch when a contraction starts. Second, she may slap your hands because she truly does not want to be touched during contractions. In this case, try massaging her between contractions and taking your hands away when a contraction starts.

Getting Yelled At

Many coaches say that they hope their partners won't yell at them during labor. Most women don't yell at their coaches, but there are exceptions. At one birth Theresa attended, the mom yelled at anyone who walked into the labor room. She didn't want medication; her primary coping technique was to be verbally abusive. It worked for her, although it wasn't fun for anyone else.

Although the men who get yelled at seldom talk about it much, a woman in labor can anger or hurt her partner by yelling at him. After all, he's doing the best he can. What should you do if your partner yells at you?

Take a deep breath. Your first response may be to yell back or to give your partner the silent treatment. These are the worst things you could do. Instead, count to five in your head, and think before you respond.

Don't take it personally. She's in pain, and her hormones are controlling her. She may need someone to verbally throw up all over, and you're an easy target.

Let her yell. Whether your partner is uncomfortable, scared, or angry about something in particular, yelling may make her feel better. Think about how much better you feel after yelling when you've stubbed your toe. You may be able to help just by being a wall she can yell at.

Try harder. Maybe she's making a point; you may not be helping her enough. Can you figure out something else for the next contraction? Pull out your cheat sheet (see page 34) and offer another position or comfort technique.

Take a break. There's only so much abuse we can take before we snap. If you're nearing the breaking point, ask another support person to help you out, or get the nurse. Go out into the hall, and count to ten.

Keeping Yourself from Fainting

Theresa remembers a dad who had planned to catch the baby; he had even taken a special class to prepare himself. The baby crowned, and the dad got his hands into position. When the baby's head was only an inch from his hands, he fainted. Luckily, the midwife was right behind him, and she caught the baby. Not only did the dad miss the moment of birth, but the peaceful scene disintegrated into chaos as staff people rushed into the room to help the dad. He'll never live it down.

Many dads are scared they'll faint during labor. Fortunately, few do. If you're concerned about the possibility, though, here's what to do:

Eat. Nothing will lead to fainting faster than going hungry for twenty-four hours in an emotionally and physically difficult situation.

Drink water. Make sure you're not getting dehydrated, especially if you're spending a lot of time with your partner in a tub or in the shower. When you're surrounded by water you may not feel thirsty, but you'll still be losing fluids. If you don't like drinking water, have some soda, Gatorade, or coffee, but avoid anything alcoholic until after the baby is born.

Rest. If your partner's labor is a long one, sheer exhaustion may make you shaky and prone to fainting. Consider calling a backup coach so you can lie down for half an hour. If your partner rests after getting an epidural, make sure you rest, too.

Listen to your body. If you get lightheaded, sit down, no matter where you are. If the lightheadedness is severe, put your head between your knees, and breathe deeply. See page 97 for some tips on preventing panic.

Avoid watching medical procedures. If your partner is getting an IV, an amniotomy (see page 110), an epidural, or a c-section, don't watch. Some dads feel comfortable viewing these procedures, but others faint at the sight of blood, needles, or other medical supplies.

Keep your head near hers. If you're afraid that the sight of the baby coming out will make you queasy, you don't have to watch. See page 27 for advice about where to stand to avoid seeing the birth.

Tell the nurse you're not feeling well. She can keep an eye on you, tell you to sit down, and give you pointers to avoid fainting.

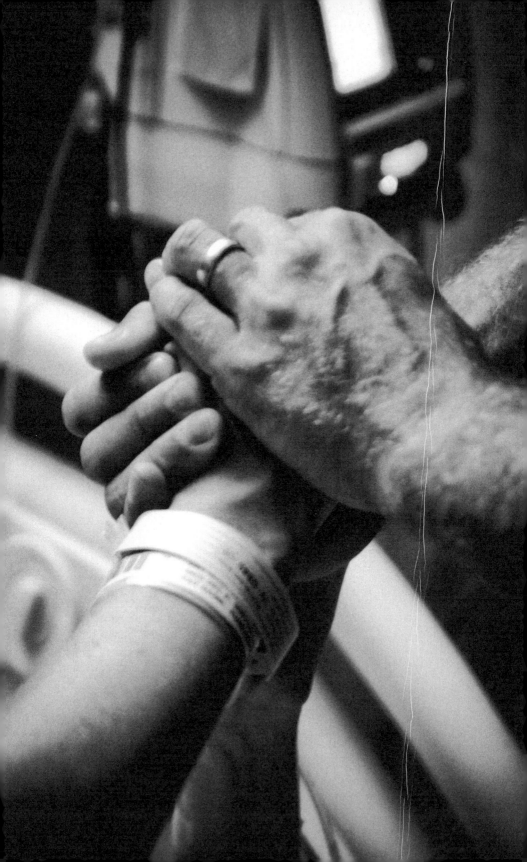

Chapter 5
TIME TO REWRITE THE PLAYBOOK: What to Do When Labor Doesn't Go as Planned

I f you've reviewed everything in Chapter 4, you're prepared for a labor that goes perfectly. But labor and childbirth rarely happen according to plan. You need to know how to deal with normal variations, such as back labor and rapid birth. You'll learn about coping with such challenges in this chapter—for instance, how to help your partner if she wants to avoid an epidural, or how to help her get one if she's sure she wants one. You'll also learn what to do during difficult obstetric procedures or if the labor ends in a cesarean birth.

Suddenly She Wants to Quit

Everything is going fine. Your partner has been coping very well with labor, and you're patting yourself on the back for being such a great coach. But then, in the space of a few contractions, she's gone from telling you that labor isn't so bad to screaming that she can't do this anymore. She wants a c-section, and she wants it now. Or she wants to go home. She's crying and saying the baby's never going to come out. Exhaustion, hunger, and emotional stress are playing with your head and hers, and nothing you try is helping. What do you do?

Remember that words have power. If she starts saying she can't go on, it's your job to convince her otherwise. As the coach, you need to motivate your player. Tell her she's doing great and the baby is fine. Remind her that labor won't last much longer. Assure her that her body knows what it's doing even if her mind doesn't. If she's asked you to use certain motivational words or phrase—for example, to tell her that she's strong or powerful—now's the time. (But prepare to duck; this may be the point at which doing exactly what you're supposed to—encouraging her—gets you hit or yelled at. Don't take her anger personally. She'll apologize after labor is over.)

Consider that this may be the end. Often, a good indication that a woman is in transition—the shortest but hardest part of labor—is the desire to quit. You might suggest a vaginal check to confirm that your partner's cervix is fully dilated. She'll feel better when she realizes that she's almost done.

Try something new. The contractions may have gotten a lot harder than she'd expected. She may need more help from you. Can you try a different massage technique or suggest a different position or breathing pattern? Would she like help getting into the shower? If you've exhausted all the tips on your cheat sheet, ask the nurse, doctor, or midwife for other ideas.

Be positive. She can't quit, and neither can you. If she's at her breaking point, you have to be strong and upbeat enough for both of you. You can have a nervous breakdown after the baby is out.

Take a break if you have to. If you're at your breaking point, ask someone else to take over. Pace the halls, go out to the parking lot and yell, or do whatever else you need to do. But don't go far. Remember that your partner may be acting this way because she's nearing the end.

She Panics

Your partner has passed beyond the point of wanting to quit. Now she's screaming, swearing, or sobbing—or all three. You can't get her to calm down and listen to you.

This situation isn't her fault or yours. Sometimes panic is just a part of labor. Tell yourself that, and do the following:

Take a deep breath. You can't help your partner if you're freaking out yourself. See page 97 for tips on how to keep from panicking.

Get her attention. Say her name, snap your fingers, clap your hands, put your face close to hers, or grab her shoulders. However you can, get her attention. (But do not slap her, as you may have seen done in some movies.)

Speak calmly and slowly. Make eye contact. Tell your partner that she's safe and doing well. If the doctor or nurse wants her to do something, slowly and calmly repeat their instructions.

Theresa once attended a birth where the mom felt the urge to push and started pushing before the doctor arrived. The nurse screamed at the mom not to push ("I'm not going to catch this baby!"). Confused by the yelling and the strong pushing contractions, the mom panicked. Her husband put his face close to hers and said gently, "Do not push. You are fine; the doctor is on the way." By repeating this over and over, he kept his partner calm until the doctor arrived, just in time to catch the baby.

 How to keep your partner from panicking One of Theresa's favorite doula tricks is this: When a mom starts to panic, ask her between contractions if she is in pain. You don't ask *during* a contraction, when you'd get an emphatic "Yes!" Between contractions, though, if your partner isn't having back labor, she shouldn't be in pain. Helping her to recognize that she's not in pain at the moment can prevent panic from even starting.

Get her to focus on her breathing. Tell her how to breathe: Say, "Breathe in . . . breathe out," or "In, two, three, four; out, two, three, four," until she gets herself under control. Or lead her in hee-hee-hee-blow breathing, as described on page 81. (If she's not panicking, though, telling her how to breathe could cause her to panic. Or to punch you in the nose.)

Remind her that contractions are short. If she's panicking because the contractions are so strong, try telling her when each contraction is peaking and when it's fading. If she's hooked up to a fetal monitor, you can see when a contraction peaks. If she's not hooked up to a monitor, figure out the rhythm of the contractions, using a clock with a second hand, so you can tell when she's about halfway through each one. You might even tell her how many breaths she needs to take before the contraction will fade.

Be forceful. If your partner is truly panicky, you may need to get bossy. Just saying, "Enough," "Calm down," "Stop crying," or "Listen to me" will probably make her focus on you and calm down. (Do not do this if she's not panicking, or she'll get really angry with you.)

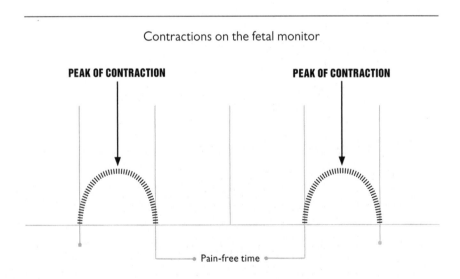

Contractions on the fetal monitor

PEAK OF CONTRACTION   PEAK OF CONTRACTION

Pain-free time

HOW TO KEEP *YOURSELF* FROM PANICKING

You know how to help your partner if she panics. But what if *you* start to panic? The key is to prevent this from happening in the first place.

- **Prepare.** Information usually helps decrease fears. By reading this book, you're learning what's normal and what's not. Taking a childbirth class and attending prenatal appointments with your partner will help, too. If you're a planner by nature, think about what you might do in certain situations (see page 6).

- **Know your triggers.** If the sight of blood makes you squeamish, you may want to look away when the baby is being born. (It's normal for a baby to come out a little bloody. The nurses usually wipe it away quickly.)

- **Take care of yourself on the big day.** It's easy to lose it if you're hungry, thirsty, exhausted, or in pain. Be sure to take time to eat and rest, if possible. If you're in pain, take painkillers. Try to prevent pain or injury by making sure you're in a comfortable position when supporting your partner. If you're not hiring a doula, consider asking someone on your support team to make sure you're taking care of yourself.

- **Take deep breaths.** If your heart is pounding, your hands are sweaty and shaking, and your knees are getting wobbly, breathe deeply. Sit down, and put your head between your legs if you're feeling you might faint. (See page 90 for more advice about preventing fainting.)

- **Leave the room if you need to.** If you're your partner's only support person, ask the nurse to stay with your partner until you get back. Go out to the hallway, walk around, and take some deep breaths to calm down.

Reassure her between contractions. After each contraction is over, remind your partner that she's feeling no pain, that you are helping her relax, and that together the two of you will deal with the next contraction. Remind her that she *can* get through labor and that you're there for her.

She Has Back Labor

Back labor is one of those things women hope they won't experience. Your partner has probably heard horror stories from family members and friends who went through it. Essentially, back labor is back pain that occurs during contractions, and it hurts much more than regular contractions. It's usually caused by the baby's posterior position, in which the back of the baby's head is pressing against the mom's back. This puts painful pressure on her joints and ligaments. The good news is that the contractions will probably make the baby rotate. The extra-good news is that you and your partner can help this process. Typically, once the baby rotates, the back pain goes away.

POSTERIOR BABY

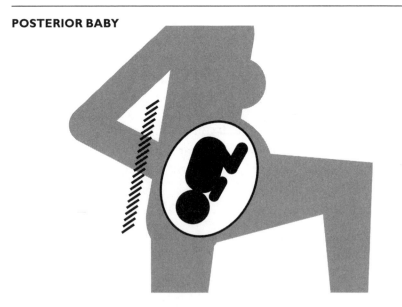

If your partner has back pain, you have two jobs: to help her get into positions that will stimulate the baby to rotate, and to help her with the pain. Luckily, there are many ways to do both.

Getting the Baby to Rotate

Have your partner try any of these positions:

Hands and knees. An all-fours position not only opens up the pelvis but also uses gravity to pull the back of the baby's head (the heaviest part of the baby) around. Usually this is the most comfortable position for moms dealing with back labor. Your partner can get in this position on the floor (on a blanket, with pillows under her knees) or on top of the bed. If she doesn't like the pressure on her wrists, she can drop to her forearms or kneel and lean on a birthing ball instead.

Lunge. Have your partner put one foot up on a sturdy chair and lunge toward the back of the chair. She'll probably put a hand on her hip, which may make you think of Captain Morgan on the rum bottle. This position opens up one side of the pelvis and stimulates the baby

---

THE LUNGE

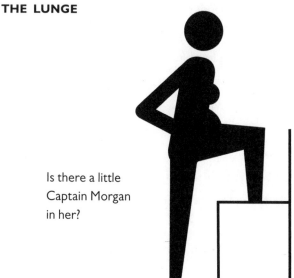

Is there a little Captain Morgan in her?

to rotate. You can lean on the back of the chair so your partner can look into your eyes, or you can stand behind her and massage her lower back.

Straddling a chair. Sitting backward in a chair opens up the pelvis, which helps the baby to rotate. This is also a great position for a back rub. Put a pillow against the back of the chair so your partner can lean forward in comfort.

Sitting on a ball. Just like straddling a chair, sitting on a birthing ball opens the pelvis and helps the contractions turn the baby around.

Helping with the Pain

While your partner is in a position that stimulates the baby to rotate, you can help her deal with the pain, in any of these ways:

Apply counterpressure. Press with your hands right where the pain is—probably in the middle of the lower back, but possibly off to one side. Use your thumbs or palms. This is a good technique to practice in childbirth class, so your instructor can help you with hand placement.

Try a rolling massage. Ever wonder why books on childbirth say to pack a tennis ball? It's for a rolling massage, which provides some relief for the lower back when a woman has back labor. You can get the same effect with a cold can of soda, a rolling pin (especially the kind you can fill with ice), or a massager with wheels.

Use heat. A favorite way to deal with back labor is with a heating pad. Try an air-activated one—you can find them in pharmacies for a few dollars. They're mildly warm, thin enough to massage through, and sticky so they stay in place. A plug-in heating pad or a rice-filled sock heated in a microwave can also help. Or you can aim the spray of hot water at your partner's lower back while she straddles a chair or birthing ball in the shower.

Try cold. If heat's not helping, cold may numb the pain. Use a cool compress or an ice pack wrapped in a towel. If the hospital doesn't provide ice packs, wrap some ice chips in a washcloth.

She's Having Uncomfortable Contractions but Not Making Progress

Here's one of the most discouraging scenarios: Your partner is having strong contractions, you've gone to your birthing facility (maybe more than once), and the nurses have sent you home because her waters haven't broken and her cervix isn't dilated enough for her to be admitted. This has gone on for many hours or even days, and you're both struggling with exhaustion and stress. Unfortunately, this situation is common enough to have a name: *prodomal labor*. What do you do about it?

Call the doctor or midwife. Ask if the care provider can recommend or prescribe anything to help your partner relax. You might have to make another trip to the hospital, but getting a sedative for your partner could help her sleep through the contractions so you can both get some rest. The care provider might instead suggest stripping your partner's membranes (see page 170) to get labor going. (Pitocin and the breaking of the water bag aren't possibilities until your partner is admitted to the hospital.)

Help your partner to relax. Treat her to a professional massage, or give her a really good massage at home. Or get her into the shower or bathtub. If she relaxes she'll be able to get some rest, and labor will be easier.

Throw away the clock. Staring at the clock makes time seem to go more slowly. Try to stop worrying about how long the process is taking, and don't time the contractions until they're obviously coming close together. Prodomal labor can last as long as a week. Just try to get through it.

Get some rest. Help her as needed during contractions, but close your eyes and try to doze between them. Yes, you will feel that the second you fall asleep she's waking you again, but you'll actually be getting a few minutes of sleep in between. Those few minutes will help you get through the next few hours or days.

Don't forget to eat. Make sure you're taking time to eat. Your partner also needs to eat, though she may have no appetite and may even throw up her food. Offer her smoothies or other flu-friendly foods, as you would in early labor (see page 56). If she won't eat, at least get her to drink, because dehydration can make contractions more painful.

Call in a backup coach. Find someone who can help your partner through contractions while you get some sleep. You may feel terrible about sleeping while she's working, but you need to get some rest to be a good coach.

Be prepared for the contractions to stop. The contractions may get closer together, raising your hopes that it's nearly time to go to the hospital, and then space back out or stop completely for a while. If this happens, enjoy the gift of rest before the contractions start up again.

She Experiences a Rapid Birth

Here's the opposite scenario: The baby comes quickly—so quickly you can't make it to the hospital in time. Although this is extremely unlikely (which is why a birth on the side of a road makes the news), here are some tips, just in case you need them.

Get to a safe place. If you're in the car and your partner starts screaming that the baby is coming, don't drive as fast as you can to the hospital. Instead, pull over, out of the way of traffic. If you're still at home, stay where you are.

Encourage your partner to blow during contractions. Most women can't push while breathing as if they're blowing a dandelion or birthday candles. Put your face close to your partner's, and tell her to blow this way until help arrives. Between contractions, have her breathe normally.

Have her change position. If you can't see the baby's head, have your partner get on her knees and forearms and drop her chest, keeping her butt up. This position will make her fight gravity to push, and so may give you a few extra minutes before the baby is born. If you can already see the baby's head, don't bother having your partner change position; it's too late.

Call for help. Call 911, and describe your situation to the dispatcher. Ask the dispatcher to send paramedics or, if you can see the baby's head, to talk you through the delivery. If you don't have time to call, yell for help, and hope someone hears and calls 911 for you.

Put the baby against Mom's bare chest. If the two of you are still alone when the baby is born, put the baby onto your partner's bare chest, and put a blanket or shirt over both of them. Your partner's body heat will keep the baby warm.

Don't worry about the umbilical cord. You could tie off the cord with a shoelace, but you don't need to. If the placenta comes out while you're still waiting for help, wrap it up, and tuck it up next to the baby.

Take a deep breath. If they haven't arrived already, paramedics should be on their way. They will transport the three of you to the nearest hospital. Or, if you still haven't called 911, call now!

She Wants an Epidural—Now!

You're in the birthing facility, your partner has been admitted, and she wanted her epidural "ten freaking minutes ago!" What do you do?

Keep her calm while she waits for anesthesia. Depending on the facility, the number of anesthesiologists available, and how many other women are waiting for cesareans or epidurals, your partner may have to wait for an hour or two before the anesthesiologist can get to her. Help her through the contractions with the information in this book, and remind her that help is on the way.

Talk with the hospital staff. Make sure that all of your partner's questions are answered and that she understands exactly what will be happening, so she won't be scared about the procedure.

Stay close by if they make you leave the room. Some hospitals have policies that require support people to leave the room during the placement of an epidural. If that's the case, stay in the hallway if the hospital allows. If they don't, go for a quick walk, make a phone call, and head back after about fifteen minutes.

Hold her as she gets the epidural. Your partner will be asked to curl into a C-shape, with her back toward the anesthesiologist or nurse-anesthetist, who will probably recommend that you stand in front of your partner. This way she can rest her head against your chest while you gently hold her head or shoulders (without touching her back). This position will help her stay still for the ten to fifteen minutes required for the anesthesiologist to place the epidural. Be aware, for some women, this position can be very uncomfortable. Stroke her head and help her breathe until the anesthesiologist or nurse-anesthetist is done. If hospital policy prevents your partner from curling into you, stay as close they will allow you. Help her breathe and focus to get through the contractions without moving.

Don't watch the procedure. Okay, okay—you can watch if you really want to. Before you look, though, ask yourself if you can handle seeing a big needle go into your partner's back. Even if you think you'll be okay, avoid looking if you're lightheaded from exhaustion or hunger, in which case you might faint. Remember, nothing would be more embarrassing than fainting while *she's* the one going through labor and delivery. We can guarantee you wouldn't hear the end of it. After the procedure, there will be a thin plastic tube coming out of your partner's back. Just seeing the tube can freak out some people, so avoid looking at it if you're squeamish.

Watch for the effects. Although an epidural can bring great pain relief, it can also have side effects (see page 13). And sometimes the pain relief is inadequate; see page 108 for tips on dealing with this.

She Really Wants to Avoid an Epidural

How about the opposite scenario? Your partner really wants to go unmedicated, and you want to help her, but labor is getting intense. You're both tired and you're starting to wonder whether she can do this without a little medical help. What should you do?

Figure out what she really wants. Some women will ask for an epidural during contractions and then change their minds between contractions. If your partner does this, she doesn't really want the epidural; she's just venting. See page 95 for advice about how to respond.

Try a different coping technique. Pull out your cheat sheet and try something new. Is there a position she hasn't used? Could you try a different massage technique? Is her back hurting? If so, use techniques for coping with back labor (see page 98). Try two contractions with the new technique. If she's still struggling, reassess the situation.

Suggest a vaginal check. Sometimes women start struggling when they're reaching the end. Learning that she's 8, 9, or 10 centimeters dilated and has only a little way to go might boost her resolve and help her avoid the epidural.

Try the shower. The shower is probably your best weapon at this point. The heat, the pressure of the spray, and the sound of the water going down the drain relaxes laboring moms. It also kills time. By the time you let your nurse know you want to try the shower, get your partner disconnected from the IV line, get her clothes off, have the monitor belt removed, turn the water on, and get the temperature right, you've already killed fifteen to thirty minutes. Your partner is that much closer to her goal. Sometimes, however, the shower is off limits—see the sidebar for more information.

Talk to the nurse, doctor, or midwife. Maybe someone can suggest a position or comfort technique you haven't tried yet. Use caution when asking for advice, though; some nurses will encourage a mom to get an epidural just because so many other women do. It's what the nurses are used to.

Consider suggesting an analgesic. An analgesic—a dose of narcotic usually given through an IV line—is an alternative to an epidural. An analgesic might help your partner relax during the contractions, and its effects would wear off in just a few hours. This might give you and your partner enough of a break for you to come up with another plan for dealing with the contractions. Make sure you and your partner learn about the pros and cons of analgesics from your childbirth educator or doctor.

Suggest that she reconsider an epidural. If she's exhausted or stressed out and doesn't want analgesics, or if she has tried them and they didn't work as she hoped they would, an epidural may be the best choice.

When walking and showering are off limits Taking a shower or walking the halls usually helps with labor, but some women find their mobility strictly limited. If there are any special concerns about the baby's condition, if your partner is having a vaginal birth after a cesarean (VBAC), or if she's on Pitocin, she will be subject to continuous fetal monitoring. Few hospitals have portable, waterproof monitors (though some do, so ask). Continuous fetal monitoring usually means close tethering to a machine. An epidural or analgesic requires not only continuous fetal monitoring but also confinement to bed.

You Both Wanted to Avoid an Epidural, But She Has Ended Up with One Anyway

If you wanted your partner to go unmedicated, you may feel she has let you down. Don't blame her. Remember, you don't know what she was experiencing. On the outside she may have been coping fine, but on the inside she may have been screaming. Here's what to do:

Support her decision. Tell her that the epidural was a good choice and that you'll continue to help her. If she experiences side effects from the epidural, remind her that she made the best decision she could make at the time. This won't be the first time she'll question a decision she has made; regrets are part of being human. And part of being a parent, too.

Let her rest. If she's been laboring for many hours or even for days, make sure she's comfortable and can sleep. You should try to get some sleep as well. See page 86 for advice on sleeping in a hospital.

When it's time for her to push, suggest having the epidural turned down or off. Many women worry, with good cause, that an epidural can make the pushing phase more difficult. To minimize this problem, you can have the epidural turned down or off when it comes time to push.

The Epidural Doesn't Work

In about 15 percent of the population, epidurals either don't provide any pain relief or don't provide enough. In addition, epidurals aren't designed to take away every sensation from the waist down, though Hollywood may make us think otherwise. With an epidural, your partner should still feel the pressure of contractions, and she may feel sensations on her perineum (see page 169) as the baby moves down. If she had been expecting completing numbness or total pain relief, she may panic when she doesn't get it. How can you help her?

Keep her calm. Tell her you'll come up with a solution. See page 95 for advice about calming a panicking mom.

Have the nurse page the anesthesiologist or nurse-anesthetist. Maybe a different medication or a bigger dose will work, or maybe the epidural catheter needs to be removed and placed again.

Support your partner as if she's going unmedicated. If the anesthesiologist or nurse-anesthetist doesn't solve the problem, pull out your cheat sheet and work your way down the list.

Ask for analgesics. A shot of narcotics may take the edge off the pain.

Suggest turning off the epidural. Lying down makes contractions much worse. If the epidural isn't providing pain relief, your partner may as well have it turned off so she can get out of bed, into an upright position, and maybe into the shower.

What if the epidural doesn't work and your partner needs a cesarean? Don't worry; doctors won't operate on a woman who can feel the surgery. In this case, the staff will probably attempt a spinal block, which is similar to an epidural but more effective. If there's no time for a spinal or it doesn't work, the staff will give your partner general anesthesia to knock her out. She'll wake up a few hours after the birth.

She Faces a Difficult Medical Procedure

Most hospitals require that laboring women at least get a saline lock (a plugged tube in a vein for quick connection to an IV line) and some labors require other medical procedures, such as internal fetal monitoring (see page 83) or an amniotomy (see page 110). Some women handle these procedures very easily, but others need their coaches' help to stay as relaxed as possible. The more relaxed the mother is, the less discomfort she'll feel. Here's what to do when the staff proposes any of these procedures.

Talk to your partner. Make sure she knows what the procedure is, what it entails, and its pros and cons. If the procedure isn't routinely required or absolutely necessary, make sure she *chooses* to have it done, rather than just accepting it. Remember what we talked about in Chapter 1: Women who don't make decisions regarding their birthing experiences are at increased risk for postpartum depression.

Talk to the staff. If they're going ahead with the procedure, let them know if your partner is nervous about it; they may make an effort to explain what they're doing or be gentler. Tell them also if your partner has had problems with the same procedure before—for example, if her IVs are hard to place.

Remind her to breathe during the procedure. Breathe with her if necessary.

Give her a focal point. Make eye contact with her, or make sure she can see whatever focal point she has been using in the room. If she prefers to close her eyes, that will help, too.

Ask the staff to stop what they're doing during a contraction. They may be able to wait while she moves, breathes deeply, or makes sounds to help her through the contraction.

She Has an Amniotomy

Many women have their bag of waters broken to start or speed up labor. In this procedure, called an amniotomy or AROM (artificial rupture of the membranes), the care provider inserts a small plastic hook into the mother's birth canal to pop the bag of waters surrounding the baby. The hook, called an amnihook, looks like a flat crochet hook or a long flat toothbrush with a very small hook rather than bristles at the end. This procedure calls for its own set of coaching instructions.

Support your partner in the usual ways. Hold her hand, have her focus on her breathing, suggest she close her eyes or gaze into yours. The breaking of the water bag won't hurt if she doesn't tense up, though it may feel strange.

Get ready for intense contractions. Breaking the bag of water causes the baby's head to drop and press directly on the cervix. Unless your partner has an epidural, this will make labor harder, and so will lying in bed, which the doctor or midwife may require for a time. Find out when your partner can get up and whether in the meantime you can raise the top of the bed to bring her into a more upright position.

Be prepared for leaks. The staff will place a plastic-lined pad on the bed to catch the first gush. More fluid will probably leak out when your partner moves or has a contraction. If this bothers her, suggest that she put on underwear and a menstrual pad.

Let the nurse know if the fluid changes color. Amniotic fluid is usually clear, but it will turn brownish or greenish if the baby has a bowel movement (see below). This is a sign that the baby is getting a little stressed.

The scoop on meconium Meconium is the baby's first poop. Most babies wait until they're born to pass it. But some get a little stressed out before they're born and pass it early. You'll know your baby has pooped if your partner's amniotic fluid looks yellow, brown, or green. There's a slight risk that the baby might inhale some amniotic fluid as he takes his first breath. If this happens after he has pooped, meconium can get into his lungs and make him very sick.

If there's meconium in the amniotic fluid, the doctor or midwife will suction out the baby's nose and mouth as soon as the head is out. When the rest of the baby's body slips out, the baby will be taken to the warmer, where the staff will suction more fluid out of the baby's nose and mouth. This might look a little scary, but it's for your baby's safety. Feel free to go over to the warmer and say hi to your baby. As soon as your baby is breathing well, he'll be placed against your partner's chest.

She Has a Cesarean

Many women attempt a vaginal birth only to have it end in a cesarean. Although the decision to operate may come as a relief—because labor is nearly over and the baby is almost here—your support duties are far from done at this point.

Accompany your partner to the operating room. In most hospitals a support person is allowed in the surgical room except in an emergency, when the mother is given general anesthesia (knocked out). If you have to wait outside, ask the doctor where you should go so you can see your partner and your baby as soon as possible after the birth.

Bring along another support person, if possible. Some hospitals allow only one support person at a cesarean, but others allow two. Having two is ideal: One can focus on Mom's emotional needs after the baby is born, so she doesn't feel forgotten, while the other focuses on the baby. If your hospital allows only one supporter in the room, ask if another can take your place if the baby has to go to the nursery or the neonatal intensive-care unit (NICU).

Avoid looking. Your partner will have a drape or screen placed over her chest to keep her from seeing what's going on, but you'll be able to watch the process, if you want to. But remember that this is major surgery, involving scalpels, blood, and organs. You might take a quick look when the baby is pulled out, but otherwise you should avoid looking. This is most important if you feel lightheaded from exhaustion or hunger; you might faint.

Stay close to your partner's face. Ask the nurse for a chair so you can rest—and to prevent you from seeing what's going on during the surgery. Hold your partner's hand. Talk to her through the procedure if it seems to calm her; make sure she understands what's going on. Feel free to ask the anesthesiologist questions. Anesthesiologists are usually good about explaining things during surgery.

Ask about taking still pictures or a video. Most hospitals have strict rules against filming surgery, but many allow still pictures of the baby immediately afterward. If the baby is rushed off to the NICU before your partner has had a good look at him, take a lot of digital pictures of the baby in the NICU and show them to Mom on your camera while she's recovering from the cesarean.

Let your partner know that she and the baby will be fine, *if you're sure that this is true*. If your partner is having a cesarean because the baby isn't doing so well, tell her that you don't know what's going to happen, but that you're with her and the two of you will get through this.

Hold your baby as soon as possible. If your baby's doing fine after the birth, ask the staff if you can hold her. Bring the baby close to your partner's face. Ask if Mom can touch the baby or give her a kiss. Unfortunately, your partner won't be allowed to hold the baby until the surgery is complete, thirty to forty minutes after the baby is born.

Decide whether to go with the baby or stay with Mom. Some hospitals separate the mom and baby while the surgery continues. This usually means that the baby goes to the recovery room or the nursery. Now you have a hard choice—do you stay with your partner or go with the baby? Ideally, you'll have talked about this possibility with your partner ahead of time and arranged for the help of another support person, if your hospital allows it.

Be there for Mom and the baby afterward. This seems obvious. But if the labor was long, your instinct may be to take a nap. Try to wait until Mom and the baby are asleep before getting some rest yourself.

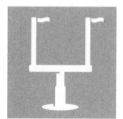

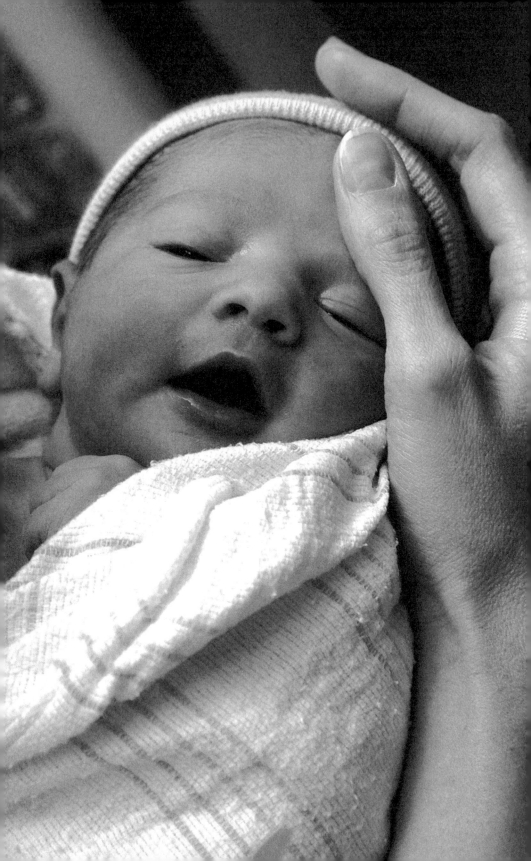

Chapter 6
HERE'S BABY! How to Help During Birth and the First Few Days

You're through the longest and, for many women, the hardest part of labor. Take a deep breath of relief. But now, epidural or no, you have to support your partner through the pushing and birth. After that, of course, there's also caring for the baby, helping with breastfeeding, and learning how to help while your partner and baby are in the hospital.

Helping with Pushing

Pushing can take just a few minutes or several hours. A lot of people think that the bigger the baby, the longer and harder the pushing will be. Though size does matter, it's not the only factor (hmm . . . where have we heard that before?). The amount of time and effort required to push a baby out also depends on the baby's position in your partner's pelvis, the size of your partner's pelvic outlet (which has nothing to do with the width of her hips), the positions she uses for pushing, whether she has an epidural, and whether this is the first baby to pass through her pelvis. Pushing out a baby is like one of those puzzles that you can't solve until you get the angles of the pieces just right, so they finally slide apart.

There's a lot you can do to help during the pushing phase. In fact, for you as well as for your partner, this may be the most physically strenuous part of labor.

Hold a leg. The two most common positions for hospital birth, side-lying and semi-sitting, require holding one or both of the mom's legs up to keep her pelvis open. (Most hospital beds have stirrups for supporting the mother's feet, but these usually aren't pulled out except for delivering the placenta and stitching the perineum, when necessary.) If your partner has an epidural, she will need extra help keeping her legs up, because they will feel very heavy and hard to control.

When you're holding your partner's legs, keep them slightly bent so you don't injure her knees, and low enough that you don't overextend them (if she's had an epidural and you find you can lift her leg up to her ear, you may be hurting her; she just doesn't know it because she's numb).

Keep her comfortable. If she's lying down, put a soft pillow behind her head. If she's lying on her side, you might put a pillow behind her back to help her rest comfortably between pushes.

Help her rest. It's very important that your partner rest between contractions. Help her get into a comfortable position. If she's squatting, make sure she can drop to her knees between pushes. You might also put a pillow in front of her to rest her head on.

Count to ten. Many care providers and nurses will count while a mom is pushing. They say something like this: "Take a deep breath in, put your chin on the chest, and push, one, two, three, four . . ." all the way up to ten. Your partner may prefer to hear your voice encouraging her, so take over the counting once you know how to do it.

Freshen cool compresses. Pushing is very hard and hot work. In between contractions, rewet compresses and move them around her body—say, from her forehead to her chest to the back of her neck. If contractions are too close together to allow for rewetting, just flip the compress over.

Fan her. If you brought a portable, battery-operated fan from home, pull it out and turn it on. Otherwise, fold a piece of paper into a fan, and start fanning. A bag that sterile gloves come in can also work well as a fan.

Offer her a drink. Keep a water bottle with a straw or spout close by. Or get a cup with a straw. Offer your partner something to drink, or ice chips to suck on, after every contraction.

Avoiding the Sight of Birth

As we discussed in Chapter 1, a lot of dads worry that the sight of the baby coming out will make them faint or vomit or will plague their minds later on. If you feel this way, hopefully you've discussed the problem with your partner ahead of time. But many men decide at the last moment whether they want to watch the baby come out. If you find yourself uncertain, ask yourself these questions:

— Does your partner want you to watch?

— Do you think the image will haunt you in the future (maybe when you're having sex or seeing your partner naked)?

— Will you be comfortable with the sight and smells of blood, amniotic fluid, urine, and poop coming out?

— Have you eaten recently? If not, you're more likely to faint at the sight of birth.

— When did you last sleep? If you've been up for longer than twenty-four hours, again, you're at more risk of fainting.

— Have you been drinking fluids? Dehydration also increases the chance of fainting.

— Has the sight of blood ever made you faint or feel lightheaded? If so, there's a good chance you're going to faint if you watch the birth.

Here's what to do if you want to stay in the room but don't want to see the birth:

Keep your eyes on your partner's face.

Ask another support person to hold a leg. When you're holding your partner's leg, you're in a perfect position to see *everything*. If you don't want to look but just can't resist, ask your partner's mom, sister, best friend, or doula to hold the leg instead.

Keep your face near your partner's. This way you'll see the baby immediately after birth, but not during the birth.

Move to the back of the room. If another support person can help your partner with cool compresses, sips of water, and so on, feel free to move away from the bed. But do this only if you've checked with your partner ahead of time.

Ask the nurse to cover your partner's lower half with a sheet. Working under a sheet will be awkward for the nurse, however.

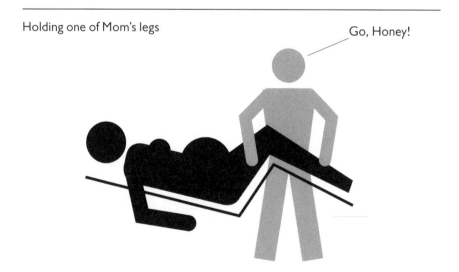

Holding one of Mom's legs

Go, Honey!

Is That the Head?

During pushing the baby's head moves in and out, appearing and disappearing. When you see a little white or gray thing coming out of your partner's parts, that's the head! As pushing progresses, the head looks odder and odder. It may be gray, blue, purple, or pink. It may have a lot of hair or no hair. It looks kind of like a walnut. You might think the baby's brains have gotten mashed up against the skull. After birth, fathers often ask how brain-damaged their babies are—that's how weird the head looks! But the wrinkly look is totally normal. It happens because the baby's skull isn't fully formed; pieces of it may overlap to help the head pass through the birth canal. This is called molding. See page 129 for more information.

 Can you catch the baby? It's unlikely that the doctor or midwife will let you, but some do allow dads to catch their babies, especially dads with medical training. It doesn't hurt to ask.

 Instrumental deliveries (with vacuum or forceps) Sometimes babies need extra helping getting out of the birth canal, either because of fetal distress (see page 166) or because Mom is too exhausted to push any longer. If this happens, the provider may use either a vacuum cap or forceps. A vacuum cap goes onto the baby's head to provide suction. It's used in 2 to 5 percent of births in this country. Forceps are metal tongs that fit around the baby's head. They are used only in extreme emergencies, in fewer than 1 percent of U.S. births. If the doctor has to use either of these tools, avoid looking; the sight can be really scary. Instead, hold your partner's hand, breathe with her, and just be there for her before and after the birth. If your baby has to go to the NICU, see page 134.

The Baby Is Here!

Your baby was just born—congratulations! Now she is placed against your partner's chest and wiped off.

APGAR Testing

If the mom and baby seem okay, this first test is done while your partner holds the baby against her chest. The doctor or midwife checks the baby's appearance (Is she pink or blue?), pulse, grimace (whether the baby makes a face or cries when rubbed with a rough cloth or tapped on the foot; this is done only if the baby is taken to the warmer because she isn't doing well), activity (Is she moving?), and respiration. The test is performed one minute after birth and again five minutes after birth. Each time, the baby gets a score between 0 and 10.

Remember, your child's APGAR score has nothing to do with how smart he is or how well he will succeed in life.

Cutting the Umbilical Cord

At this point the doctor or midwife will probably invite you to cut the umbilical cord. Don't worry; the cord doesn't have any nerves in it, so you can't hurt your partner or your baby by cutting it. It does have blood in it, though, so you may see the blood spurt when you cut the cord. It is also harder to cut than you would think; cutting it takes a little bit of strength. If you don't want to cut, you don't have to. The staff will do it for you.

Out Comes the Placenta

While you're excited about meeting your baby, your partner still has to deliver the placenta. This organ filtered blood and provided nutrients to the baby throughout the pregnancy, helping your baby grow big and strong. After the baby is born, she no longer needs the placenta, so it comes out.

After your partner has pushed out the baby, delivering the placenta will be super-easy. If she has had an epidural, she may not even know she has delivered the placenta until her care provider tells her.

If you want, the doctor or midwife will show you the placenta. Combined with the cord and amniotic sac, the placenta is a very cool organ, or so Theresa thinks. It's interesting to see where the baby lived. But Brad thinks placentas are gross and doesn't know why someone would want to look at one. Chances are you'll be so focused on your baby that you won't care much about the placenta.

Until, maybe, your partner says she wants to take it home. Many couples choose to take the placenta home, for various reasons, including to eat it (see the sidebar). You could bury the placenta in your yard and plant a tree over it, make it into jewelry (yes, some people do), press it onto a piece of paper to make an art print, or just stick it in your freezer for a while. Theresa even saw one placenta that had been dried and sewn into the shape of a bear (hey, no throwing up on this book!).

You have the right to bring the placenta home, but some hospitals are difficult about this, so be sure to ask ahead. Bring along a big Tupperware container, and be prepared to sign some extra papers.

If you don't want to take the placenta home, the hospital will be happy to incinerate it for you.

Why would anyone eat a placenta? Although no research has yet confirmed this, some people swear that eating the placenta after birth prevents postpartum depression and exhaustion. You can cook placenta into many foods (pizza, cakes, smoothies—no throwing up!), or a professional can clean and dry it, grind it into powder, and pack the powder into capsules for your partner to take every couple of hours in the first few weeks.

Your Partner's Privates After Birth

After your partner delivers the placenta, you may notice the doctor or midwife doing some additional work on your partner's perineum (see page 169) and birth canal. The care provider is checking for tears, which sometimes require stitches. Don't look! The sight might be upsetting for you, and you should be focusing on your partner and your baby anyway. Your partner won't feel the stitching, because if she hasn't had an epidural she'll have gotten a numbing shot, or several. (If she *does* feel the stitching, tell the doctor or midwife.) If your partner has had an episiotomy (see page 166), the process may take a while. Just help your partner focus on the baby. The provider is working as fast as possible.

Because the stitches are the kind that dissolve over time, they won't have to be removed. But the provider may give your partner some instructions to follow to prevent irritation and infection, such as using a squirt bottle of warm water instead of toilet paper after peeing and forgoing sexual intercourse for a few weeks (see page 142). Before you leave the hospital, make sure your partner understands the instructions.

Depending on the amount of repair that's needed, your partner may be sore for the next few days or weeks. She may need some help when she stands up or sits down. She may need to sit on a special pillow to take pressure off her perineum. She may also be need to take ibuprofen (such as Advil) or acetaminophen (such as Tylenol), both of which are safe during breastfeeding.

When Do You Get to Hold Your Baby?

The baby may go over to the warmer for a quick evaluation, but then she'll come back to your partner. You kiss your partner, tell her how amazing she is, and take some pictures (if you're the cameraman). Now your partner is holding and kissing the baby, and you're wondering when you get a turn.

Wait a good hour. If your partner is going to be breastfeeding, try to hold off asking to hold the baby. When many people handle a baby right after birth, the baby can get a little overwhelmed and may not nurse as well during the first breastfeeding session. And that first session is very important. The better it goes, the higher the chance that the baby will continue to nurse well. After the first hour and the first nursing, you can hold the baby. And don't let grandmas or aunts muscle you out. The first person to hold the baby after Mom and the doctor or midwife should be you!

Keep Mom calm. If breastfeeding is going to get off to a good start, Mom needs to be calm. The thing that stresses out moms the most is people running around and asking questions. If friends and relatives are waiting in the lobby for news about the baby, make them wait a little longer. If these people are already in the room, kick them out. Tell them that you need some family time and that they can meet the baby later.

Keep the baby calm. An upset baby won't breastfeed well. He may also have trouble making the transition from a water environment to an air environment (see the section on APGAR testing). This can mean a trip to the NICU for observation, which would be upsetting for you and your partner. Make sure your partner is holding the baby against her bare chest. The familiar sound of Mom's heartbeat, her smell, her voice, and her touch will all help keep the baby calm. Your touch and your voice will also calm the baby, who knows your voice almost as well as he knows your partner's.

Skin-to-skin contact Babies who are held skin-to-skin immediately after birth—bare against the mother's bare skin—generally have better body temperatures, better heart rates, better respiration, and better blood sugar levels. These babies also tend to breastfeed sooner and longer.

Your holding the baby skin-to-skin can have almost the same benefits as your partner's doing it, except where breastfeeding is concerned. Skin-to-skin contact has been shown to have benefits throughout a baby's first year. Babies frequently held this way bond with their parents better, breastfeed better, and cry less.

Baby security If your partner has delivered in a hospital, your baby will have a security band fastened to his ankle within moments of birth. You and your partner will get matching bands. These bands are for your baby's protection; if your baby is sent to the nursery, the bands may beep if a nurse tries to hand you the wrong baby. The hospital will probably also have cameras and alarms set up in hallways and doorways to prevent baby theft. Your doctor or midwife can tell you more about the hospital's security policies.

Newborn Procedures

Within an hour or two after birth, the staff will bathe, weigh, and measure your baby and perform a few newborn medical procedures. Some nurses and doctors want to do these procedures immediately after birth, but you might ask the staff to wait an hour or two, as the procedures can interfere with bonding and breastfeeding.

— Vitamin K shot. This helps your baby's blood to clot, to reduce the risk of a rare but serious bleeding condition.

— Erythromycin ointment. This antibiotic goes into the baby's eyes to eliminate the risk of a potentially blinding eye infection.

— Newborn screening tests. Samples of the baby's blood are taken. These samples will be tested for rare genetic and metabolic disorders that are treatable if caught early.

Helping with Breastfeeding in the Hospital

Sometime after your baby is placed against your partner's bare chest, you may see your baby do a commando-wiggle over to a breast, wag her head around like a bobblehead in search of the nipple, and attach herself. Mom might like to support the baby's bottom and aim her breast into the baby's mouth, but she really doesn't have to. All healthy mammals have an inborn desire and ability to find and suck from their mothers' nipples after birth. Dr. Christina Smillie calls this process Baby-Led Breastfeeding.

The first breastfeeding session may happen a little differently in your hospital. The nurse may hurry the process along so she can fill out her chart and move on to other patients. In this case, she'll grab your partner's boob in one hand and the baby in the other. Then she'll tickle the baby's lips with your partner' nipple until the baby opens wide (keep your fingers crossed!), and shove the baby onto the boob. The baby may start sucking immediately—or not.

If your partner wants to try Baby-Led Breastfeeding, you may have to ask the nurse to back off. You might give the baby a half hour to show some interest in nursing before letting the nurse help get the baby onto the breast.

Hopefully you and your partner will have taken a breastfeeding class or spoken with a lactation educator or the doctor or midwife about the first nursing session and how it goes in your birthing facility. Your partner may want to read a whole book on the subject of breastfeeding, but here are a few general tips for you, so you can help your partner and baby get breastfeeding off to a good start.

Breastfeeding in a nutshell For the first few days after the birth, your partner will produce a thick, highly nutritious milk called colostrum. This early milk, full of fats and antibodies, is exactly what your newborn needs. And the tablespoon he gets at each feeding is plenty to fill up his stomach, which is the size of a shooter marble. He doesn't need anything else.

Your partner's mature milk will come in between the third and fifth days after birth, if she's been breastfeeding a lot. (If she's had a c-section or epidural, her milk is likelier to come in closer to day 5 than day 3.) The breast works according to the law of supply and demand: If your partner nurses the baby or pumps her milk frequently, she should produce plenty. If instead she stops breastfeeding or feeds a lot of formula in the early weeks, her milk supply will dwindle away.

Keep the room calm. A tense mother has a tense baby, since the baby picks up on the moods of her caregivers. A tense baby won't breastfeed well. So you need to keep your partner and the baby calm and free from distractions. This may mean kicking people out, especially if your partner's not comfortable breastfeeding in front of them (Theresa wouldn't nurse in front of her father, brothers, or father-in-law). You might also dim the lights and put on some soft music.

Expect your partner to spend a lot of time breastfeeding. She should be nursing every two to three hours, or eight to twelve times a day, unless the baby's doctor or a lactation consultant says otherwise. In the early weeks, each feeding should take about thirty to sixty minutes.

Avoid artificial nipples, if possible. Some dads can't wait to feed their babies, but pacifiers and bottles can confuse new babies and cause them to struggle with breastfeeding. In addition, feeding formula could interfere with your partner's milk supply. Unless your baby is in the NICU, it's best to wait until she is four weeks old and nursing well before introducing a bottle or pacifier.

Feeding cues Long before a baby starts crying of hunger, he'll quietly signal that he's ready for a meal. Feeding cues include increased alertness, tongue movements, sucking on a hand or fist, and rooting—turning his head toward a chest and trying to latch on. Your baby may root toward anyone holding him, including his grandma, the nurse, and you.

Get an expert's help. If your hospital has a lactation consultant, ask to have her visit your partner. A nurse with advanced training in lactation might be able to help your partner get the baby latched on, answer basic questions, and troubleshoot minor problems. But if you have multiples or a sick baby, our best advice is to see a lactation consultant, even if this means hiring one privately. Check the website of the International Lactation Consultant Association (ILCA.org) to find one in your area.

Make sure your baby stays with Mom. If your baby goes to the nursery, he'll come back crying with hunger. A baby who is crying for food is very frustrated. If the baby stays at Mom's side instead, she can put him to the breast as soon as he starts showing feeding cues (see the sidebar above).

What If Your Baby Is Ugly?

Newborns don't look like Gerber babies. We remember showing off pictures of our sons to friends who obviously lied when they said our babies were cute. Theresa was hurt, until a couple of years later when she looked at the pictures and realized that her beautiful newborn sons looked like baby monkeys. They were born early, but even full-term babies are usually kind of ugly.

Here's a list of normal newborn characteristics that can make a baby unattractive.

— **Mongolian spots.** Some African-American and Asian babies have dark patches of skin on their lower backs and butts. These fade within a year and don't mean anything.

— **Pale skin.** If you've been expecting a dark-skinned baby, you may be surprised by how pale your baby is. Don't fret; she really is your baby. Her skin tone will darken over the next few weeks.

— **Stork bites.** Raised patches of blood vessels on the face, shoulders, and back of the neck are normal on some babies. These usually fade within a couple of years.

— **Lanugo hair.** Fine hair on the back, cheeks, and shoulders makes some babies look like monkeys or gorillas. This hair rubs off over the first few weeks.

— **Skinniness.** Newborns often look scrawny. Your baby will probably have pudgy cheeks within a few weeks.

— **Vernix.** This creamy, cottage-cheese-like stuff covers the baby before birth, to protect the skin from the amniotic fluid. Babies born early have a lot of vernix; more mature babies have vernix only in skin folds and behind the ears. Vernix is either absorbed into the skin or washed or rubbed off.

— **Swollen genitals and breasts.** Most boys are born with swollen, reddened scrotums. Most newborn girls have swollen genitals, too, and some even produce a few drops of menstrual-like blood in the diaper. Both male and female babies usually also have swollen breasts, which may even produce a tiny bit of milk. All of these things are normal. They are caused by a surge of hormones from Mom at birth.

— **Smooshed nose or ears.** Many babies have ears or noses that are bent out of shape for a few days after birth, because of pressure during the passage through the birth canal.

— **Cone head.** If your baby is born vaginally, you may notice that his head isn't symmetrical. In fact, his head may even be slightly pointed. This cone shape is caused by the molding of the skull as it passes through the birth canal. Because the baby's skull bones aren't fully formed, they can overlap to help the head fit through. Keep a hat on your baby's head if the point bothers you. It should go down in a few days.

— **Milia.** These baby zits look exactly like whiteheads, and each may be surrounded by a patch of red skin. They will clear up without treatment within a few weeks. Don't apply zit cream, and don't pop these zits. You might hurt your baby and cause a scar.

The Day in the Hospital
After a Vaginal Birth

After a vaginal birth, your partner and baby will probably stay in the hospital for twelve to twenty-four hours. You may be allowed to stay with them, or you may have to leave at night (page 132). What should you be doing during the hospital stay?

Limit visitors. Theresa has heard it over and over: The visitors weren't so bad during the birth, but after the baby came everyone showed up. It's best to establish guidelines for visitors before the baby arrives. Too many can affect Mom's health, the baby's health, your stress levels, and even your partner's milk supply. Again, you may have to ask people to leave.

Make sure your partner gets time to rest. She has just gone through a physically demanding experience, and her body is very tired. It's hard for her to rest when there are people in the room whom she feels she has to entertain.

Remind her to eat and drink. She needs to replace fluids she lost during the birth. Drinking plenty of fluids (especially cranberry juice) will also help prevent bladder infections, which are common in women who have had urinary catheters (and most women who have epidurals get urinary catheters). Eating nutritious foods, especially those high in iron, such as lean red meat and leafy greens, will give her energy and help her feel better.

Feeding your partner in the hospital If your partner has been missing specific foods that she couldn't eat in pregnancy, like soft cheese or sushi, consider going out to fetch some while she's in the hospital or ask a friend to bring some in. If she hates the hospital food, consider bringing her *anything* else to eat. When Theresa was in the hospital on bed rest, Brad had a pizza delivered for her.

Help her move. Depending on what happened during labor and delivery, she may need help getting to the bathroom, sitting upright, or moving over to a chair for breastfeeding.

Fill any prescriptions. Your partner's doctor may prescribe a pain-killer or other medication. Pick up the medicine before it's time to leave the hospital, so your partner and the baby don't have to wait in the pharmacy.

Help with paperwork. The two of you will have to fill out applications for a birth certificate and Social Security card and other forms before your baby and partner can leave. See if you can take care of the paperwork so she can focus on taking care of the baby.

Learn how to care for the baby. If you've never changed a diaper, dressed a baby, or taken a rectal temperature, now's your chance. Practice this stuff in the hospital, where a nurse can help you.

Play nice with any roommates. Depending on your hospital, your partner may end up with a roommate or two. Try to respect them. One of Theresa's worst memories of her birth experience was of a roommate who arrived at 2:00 A.M. with nine other people, all of them celebrating the birth of the baby. Our own babies were in the NICU (page 134), and Theresa was trying to recover from a c-section. Despite the nurse's repeated requests, these people would not be quiet.

What if the hospital kicks you out at night? If your partner is in a shared room, the hospital will probably enforce visiting hours, which means you'll be asked to leave at night.

You may feel horrible about this, but at least you'll be able to get some rest so you'll be ready to help your partner once she and the baby come home. Get some sleep, take a shower, and have something to eat. Depending on the hospital, the baby, the nurses, and any roommate, your partner may have a restful night, sleeping between feedings, or she may get no sleep at all. In the morning, she may be counting the minutes until you're back. Consider bringing her some flowers or another small gift.

The Days in the Hospital After a C-section

If your partner has had a c-section, she'll stay in the hospital for two to four days, depending on the hospital's policy, your health insurance, your partner's health, and the baby's health. She'll need more help from you than she would after a vaginal birth, because a c-section is major surgery. Although she'll be very tired, she'll still need to wake up to feed the baby every two to three hours. What can you do to help?

Help her get up and move around. Although this may seem counterintuitive, walking around will actually help decrease her pain. But it will be difficult for your partner to go from lying to sitting and from sitting to standing. As much as you can, be around to help.

Talk to her doctor about food. There is a great deal of debate in the medical community about eating after a c-section. Some providers feel that women should have only liquids, gelatin, and juice bars until their bowels are working (until they fart). Other providers allow women to eat solid foods as soon as they feel ready. Current research backs up the second practice.

Keep everything she needs within reach. Because it is so difficult for her to get up, you'll want to make sure she can reach whatever she needs. If the baby is sleeping in a bassinet, you'll need to help her get the baby out when he wakes to feed.

Remind her to take her pain meds. Many women avoid taking pain medicine after a c-section because they're concerned the medicine will get into the breast milk. It's true that traces will reach the milk, but it's important that your partner take the medication anyway. Not only will she be more comfortable and better able to rest between feedings, but she'll prevent pain from interfering with the hormone cycle that brings in mature milk. As lactation consultants say, it's better to have milk with trace amounts of pain medicine than no milk at all.

Keep her calm if her milk comes in late. Even if your partner has been taking her pain meds, her mature milk will probably come in later than average, around day 5. She will very likely be anxious about this. Encourage her to keep breastfeeding every two hours to help trigger the hormones that start the production of mature milk.

Watch for signs of postpartum depression. Women who have c-sections are more likely to get depressed, especially if they had their heart set on giving birth vaginally. See page 144 for the symptoms of postpartum depression.

When Your Baby Goes to the NICU

However dreadful the thought, every birth brings the possibility that the baby will be sent to the neonatal intensive-care unit, or NICU. The NICU is a nursery specially designed for the needs of sick babies. Your baby may go there for brief observation, or she may need to stay for some time. What do you do if your baby is sent to the NICU?

Visit your baby. Experts agree that the more time parents spend with their babies in the NICU, the better the babies do. If you live far from the hospital, talk to the staff. They may be able to suggest a hotel with a special rate for patients' families, a place to rent an RV, or a Ronald McDonald House (a charitable "home away from home" for families of hospitalized children).

Call to check on your baby. During the night, or whenever you and your partner aren't at the hospital, feel free to call and talk to a nurse about how your baby is doing. You won't be bothering the nurses; they're used to this. Checking in frequently may help you and your partner feel better.

Take care of your baby. When our sons were in the hospital, we helped with diaper changes, feedings, and temperature taking. We also simply held the babies to keep them calm and content. If your baby is healthy enough for skin-to-skin contact (see page 124), wear a button-down shirt into the NICU so you can unbutton it to cuddle your baby rather than taking it off completely.

Keep calm and quiet. Sick babies need little light and a lot of quiet. You may be warned against taking flash pictures or talking loudly in the NICU. The hospital will also insist on keeping visitors to a minimum.

Learn and stick to hospital policies. There will be other policies to follow; for example, you'll be required to wash your hands when you come into the NICU and before handling the baby. Talk with the staff if you don't understand a policy or the reason for it.

Get help with housework and other chores. Your partner's job is to care for the baby. If the baby isn't able to breastfeed, your partner will be pumping her breast milk around the clock. Friends and family members probably won't be hanging around while the baby is in the NICU, so you may need to ask for their help with food and chores.

One of the best gifts we received when our sons were in the NICU was a full meal from some friends—chicken, rice, a fruit salad, and homemade bread. It was the first meal we'd had since the birth that wasn't fast food or a microwaved frozen meal. We felt much better going back to the hospital afterward.

Process your own emotions. If your baby is sick and can't come home with you, allow yourself to feel sad and scared. See page 144 for more information about daddy depression.

Breast milk for a baby in the NICU If your baby isn't yet breastfeeding, he still needs your partner's milk. If he was born prematurely, your partner's body will try to compensate through her milk. Mothers of premature babies produce milk with more antibodies, calories, and nutrition than the milk of other mothers. But the milk must be pumped out and fed by hand.

Make sure your partner has all of the supplies she needs and plenty of time to pump. You might find out how to rent a hospital-grade pump, and help make sure that each container of breast milk is labeled with the date and time, refrigerated, and transported to the hospital. You might also help by cleaning the pump parts, as Brad did for Theresa after every single pumping session. Finally, ask if you can help feed your baby the pumped breast milk.

The circumcision decision We won't take a stand for or against circumcision, but we will say that, at this time, the American Academy of Pediatrics maintains that the medical benefits of the procedure fail to outweigh the risks. The majority of U.S. parents who have their sons circumcised do so for cosmetic or religious reasons. Because insurance companies consider circumcision a cosmetic procedure, they cover it only partially, if at all. If you have questions about the pros and cons of circumcision, talk with your childbirth educator, your partner's doctor or midwife, or your baby's doctor.

Many hospitals will do a circumcision before the mom and baby go home; others ask parents to make a later appointment with a pediatrician. If you want your son circumcised, you should probably have it done before the baby is thirty days old, after which age circumcision becomes a major surgical procedure requiring general anesthesia.

Because so many men have fainted while watching circumcisions, many hospitals and doctors no longer allow parents to view the procedure.

Going Home from the Hospital

Leaving the hospital can be quite an event. People will be buzzing in and out of your partner's room with papers to sign and instructions. You may think you're ready to go, but then there may be more paperwork and another bunch of questions for your partner to answer. When you're through with all that, your baby may need a diaper change or a quick feeding. Fortunately, there are a couple of things you can do to make the departure as easy as possible for all three of you:

Make multiple trips. Put the bags, pillows, birthing ball, and anything else you brought with you into the car before your partner checks out. This way you won't have to deal with the baby, your partner, bright sunlight or rain, and all your stuff, too. You can just focus on getting your baby and partner loaded into the car.

Bring the car around. Most hospitals require moms to ride to the outside door of the hospital in a wheelchair, and then to walk or be wheeled to the car. If your partner had a c-section or perineal stitching, she may find walking difficult. If possible, bring the car to the door or find a close spot in the parking lot. See page 41 about car-seat installations.

Helping the First Few Weeks

You're home from the hospital with your newborn! Here are some things you can do to make the transition as smooth as possible.

Take time off work. Depending on your state and employer, you may be able to take off several weeks after the baby is born (see page 39). If you can manage this, do it.

Let things go. Get used to it: Your house will not be clean for the next eighteen years. Bonding with your baby and making sure you and your partner are getting rest are much more important than cleaning.

In years to come, you won't remember the mess. Instead, you will remember singing to your baby, cuddling with your baby, and feeling your partner's undying love for taking care of her.

Simplify your life. Keep two piles of laundry, clean and dirty. Don't worry about folding clothes. If dishes are piling up, switch to paper plates; they may be bad for the environment, but you'll need them for only a few weeks. Don't worry about dusting or vacuuming; just bend over and pick up the pet-hair tumbleweeds. Cook simple meals. If you hate cooking, ask friends and family to bring over freshly prepared foods, or thaw out those casseroles that you and your partner froze before the baby was born.

Prioritize. If you're taking time off work, your only jobs other than taking care of the baby and your partner should be eating, showering, and brushing your teeth. Everything else can wait.

Deal with visitors. Friends and family you didn't know you had may come out of the woodwork to see your new baby. Schedule their visits so you'll have just as much help as you need when you need it. And make sure people aren't planning to "help" by holding the sleeping baby while you and your partner clean, do laundry, run errands, and cook, and then pass the baby back to you when she cries. Let visitors know you'd like them to clean and cook and so on. Then they can hold the baby as much as they'd like while you and your partner *sleep*.

Consider hiring a postpartum doula. This kind of doula comes to your house after the baby is born to help with breastfeeding and baby care and to do light chores and run errands. If you have to go to work, a doula can keep your partner company and make sure she's not getting depressed. Some doulas will even come at night to care for the baby while the parents sleep. Postpartum doulas are like grandmothers who don't judge you or carry emotional baggage. Your doctor or midwife can probably provide a referral.

Sleep deprivation If you've never been awake for forty-eight hours straight, you may have no idea what sleep deprivation can do to you. Not only does it make you feel lousy, but it also increases your chances of illness, depression, moodiness, and mental disorders. Chronic sleep deprivation can make you gain weight and age faster. There is good reason that sleep deprivation is a tool of torturers.

To minimize sleep deprivation, try to sleep while your baby sleeps. Learn to nap during the day by making the room as dark as possible. Even if you and your partner just lie down and close your eyes for a few minutes, you both will feel better afterward. If your baby cries in the middle of the night but doesn't seem hungry, take turns holding and soothing her so both you and your partner can get some sleep (while wearing earplugs).

Dad-Tips for Baby Care

If your partner is breastfeeding, you may feel she's getting all the fun time with the baby. But there are a lot of ways that you can help care for your newborn. Here are a few:

Diapering. You may be dreading this job, but it's not as bad as you probably think. If your partner is breastfeeding, the baby poop won't start smelling until you give the baby solid food or formula. Actually, diaper changes are a fun time to play with and talk to your baby. In about a week or two you'll be expert at it. Just make sure you clean all the folds and crevices and, after a big blowout, check for poop up the baby's back. If you've got a baby girl, wipe from front to back. If you have a boy, get quick at putting a washcloth or wipe over his penis, and keep your mouth closed, or be ready to duck.

Baby poop In the beginning, baby poop is thick, tarry, greenish-black meconium. Luckily, it doesn't smell bad. After a few days, breastfed babies get runny, mustard-colored poops that look seedy. Formula fed babies have thicker, smellier, more formed poops. Once you feed your baby solid foods, the poop starts changing colors. You may be able to tell what the baby has eaten by the color of her poop.

Burping. Before you leave the hospital, have a nurse show you the different burping positions—over the shoulder, sitting up, and over the knees (save the last until your baby gets good neck control). Pounding on the baby's back does not get burps out faster, so be gentle. And always remember to use a burp cloth for spit-ups, which can stain clothing.

Jiggling. Many dads get really good at soothing a baby to sleep by rocking or jiggling him. Rocking mimics your baby's experience inside your partner's tummy and calms the baby down. Just make sure you support his head while you jiggle him. If you become frustrated with your baby's crying, put him down in a safe place and walk away for a few minutes.

Enjoying your baby. You'll love watching your baby, smelling her new-baby smell, and listening to her breathe. Take at least a few minutes every day to simply enjoy your newborn, because this time won't last very long. Trust us, you'll miss it once your child is crawling, walking, throwing temper tantrums, and talking back to you.

Colic A baby who cries for three hours a day at least three times a week for three weeks is said to have colic. No one knows what causes this condition, which usually peaks at six weeks and is gone by three months. A baby with colic is more likely to be shaken (sometimes hard enough to cause brain damage), and parents of colicky babies are more likely to become depressed and have problems with their relationship. If your baby has colic, talk to her doctor, who can run some tests and suggest ways to cope.

Helping with the Breastfeeding at Home

The American Association of Pediatrics recommends that babies be exclusively breastfed for six months and that breastfeeding should continue through at least the first year. If your partner feels she needs professional assistance with nursing, you might help her find a lactation consultant through the International Lactation Consultant Association (ILCA.org). For minor problems, you might hire a postpartum doula. Whether or not your partner gets help from the pros, there are a lot of things you can do to ensure that breastfeeding goes well at home:

Help your partner get comfortable. In the beginning, most women choose a specific place to breastfeed, usually a couch, rocking chair, or upholstered armchair. Make sure your partner always has at hand a pillow to put beneath the baby, another to put behind her back, and a footstool, if possible.

Bring her things. Once she's settled in to breastfeed, your partner may not be able to get up for thirty to sixty minutes. Breastfeeding makes some women thirsty and hungry, so your partner may need you to bring her water and snacks.

Help with nighttime feedings, if possible. You might bring the baby to your partner for a feeding, go back to sleep, and then wake up to burp the baby and change his diaper when the feeding is done. Even if you've gone back to work, you might still try to help with one feeding each night. Go to bed a little earlier, if possible, to ensure that you get enough sleep.

Sex After the Baby Arrives

Now that your partner is no longer pregnant, you're starting to get that feeling. You're wondering, when can we have sex again? Sex is an important part of your relationship, but most doctors and midwives want couples to postpone it for at least four to six weeks, until the lochia (see page 167) stops, any perineal tears are healed, and Mom feels ready.

Here are some things you should know before you ask whether your partner is interested:

You should use contraception. In one of Mother Nature's nasty tricks, many women become fertile soon after having a baby—sometimes even more fertile than before. This means that your partner may be able to get pregnant the first time she has sex after giving birth, even if she's exclusively breastfeeding. How happy do you think she'll be if she gets pregnant six weeks after having a baby?

There are plenty of choices among contraceptive methods. Even some hormonal options, like the minipill, are safe for breastfeeding women (if your partner is nursing, she'll want to avoid any pill containing estrogen, which could reduce her milk supply). You could instead use a good ol' condom or another barrier method. If your partner used a diaphragm or cervical cap before getting pregnant, she'll need her size rechecked.

You'll need to go slow and be imaginative. Many women are sore for several weeks or even months after giving birth. Certain positions or even intercourse itself may be out of the question, though activities of other sorts might satisfy both of you (wink, wink, nudge, nudge).

You may need a good lubricant. Breastfeeding women often need a lubricant during sex. Many options are available, including flavored and warming ones for extra fun.

Her breasts may leak. Or they may spray dramatically. If your partner is embarrassed about this or you don't like getting squirted in the face, she should feed the baby before you get busy or simply wear a sexy bra.

She may feel "touched out." If your partner is breastfeeding, she has a baby attached to her for several hours a day. When she has her body to herself for more than a few minutes, she may not look forward to cuddling or even hand holding.

Her libido will be reduced for a while. It usually takes several months for a woman's hormones to get her back in the mood. Be patient. Candles, chocolates, massages, other gifts, and romantic dinners may help.

Sleep is a priority. For the first few months after the birth, sleep is a higher priority than sex for both of you. When your baby is sleeping more at night, you and your partner will get in the mood more often.

You have to communicate. You may be ready, but she may not be. Or maybe she's ready, but you need a little more time. That's fine—when you're ready, just let your partner know. If she's not ready, wait a while and then check again.

You will have sex again A couple Brad and Theresa know didn't have sex for a full year after their baby's birth. He was worried that she wasn't ready, and she was worried that he was traumatized by seeing the baby come out. When they finally talked about the problem, they realized that they had both been waiting for the other to initiate things. Don't let this happen to you. Sex is an important part of your relationship.

Baby Blues, in Moms and Dads

In the first few weeks after the birth, both you and your partner may feel sad, anxious, moody, stressed, and irritated. Your partner may be crying for no reason and acting mildly depressed, much as she may have done in the past just before her period started. You may feel out of control and unhappy, and you both may have sleeping and eating problems. If so, you have the baby blues. The baby blues are caused by sleep deprivation, changes in your life, and hormonal shifts, possibly in both of you. To get some relief, focus on the baby, try to get more sleep, exercise, neglect unnecessary chores, and allow others to help.

The baby blues normally disappear after the first few weeks. If they don't, one or both of you may have moved into postpartum depression.

Postpartum Depression, in Moms and Dads

Some dads as well as moms get postpartum depression. Watch out for these symptoms in either of you:

— Feeling down, angry, or worthless most or all of the time

— Crying a lot more than normally (this occurs less often in men)

— Physical symptoms such as headaches, backaches, and stomach problems

— Sleeping much of the time, or not sleeping

— Eating too much, or lacking appetite

— Feeling detached from the baby

— Fatigue

— Difficulty making decisions or concentrating

You're at a higher risk for postpartum depression if any of the following are true:

— Your partner has postpartum depression.

— The baby wasn't planned.

— The birth didn't go as you or your partner had hoped.

— The baby has health problems.

— You aren't the biological father.

— You have a family history of depression or other mood disorders.

— You're having problems with your job, your finances, or other personal matters.

In rare cases after a birth, a woman hears voices or loses touch with reality. This is called postpartum psychosis. If your partner experiences this, call a doctor immediately.

Preventing or Dealing with Postpartum Depression

If you suspect you or your partner has postpartum depression, call a doctor. The longer you wait, the worse the depression may get. Postpartum depression is treatable, with therapy, antidepressants (if needed), and the following measures, which may help both of you avoid depression in the first place.

Eat healthy foods. Plenty of whole grains, fruits, vegetables, dairy products, and lean meats will help both of you feel more energetic and even-tempered.

Get some exercise. If you can't make it to the gym, try to take a family walk most days of the week. Or run or bike every day, if only for five to ten minutes. If you truly can't exercise, at least go outdoors for a few minutes of sunlight each day. Sunlight can help relieve depression.

Try to get more sleep. Repeat it with us: *Sleep when your baby sleeps.* If your baby has colic (see page 141), split sleep shifts with your partner, and use ear plugs if you have to. Take daytime naps if you can. If it's hard for you to get to sleep in the daytime, darken the room as much as possible, or use an eye mask (available at a pharmacy or online).

Let things go. Unless they have a maid or a lot of help from friends or relatives, Theresa becomes very concerned about how a couple is coping with parenthood if their house is totally clean soon after the birth of a baby. A clean house can mean that someone is cleaning rather than sleeping. Use shortcuts (like paper plates to cut down on dishwashing) whenever possible. Remember, your house won't be clean for the next eighteen years. For your sanity and your partner's, learn to live with the mess. You're not going to look back at this period and wish you'd had more cleaning time instead of baby time.

Take time off from work. Try to take off several weeks after your baby is born. Talk with your employer about going on disability, using vacation time, or working part-time. Your partner should take off as much time as her employer (and your budget) allow.

Talk with your partner. Let her know how you're feeling. She may be feeling the same way. If she needs to talk to you about her feelings, listen. When people talk about their feelings, they usually feel better afterward.

Talk with other parents. They know what you're going through. Talk with friends and coworkers who are parents, or join a daddy group and suggest that your partner join a mommy group. If there aren't such groups in your area, consider starting one. Your childbirth educator or your doula may be able to give you advice about this.

Take time for yourself. You probably shouldn't try to go out every weekend with your friends, but both you and your partner can do some of the fun things you did before your baby was born. You're not a jerk for going to a poker game or a sporting event, or playing golf once or twice a month after your baby is born. Just make sure Mom also has chances to do some fun shopping (not at the grocery store!) or go on an occasional girls' night out.

Make dates with your partner. At least once a month, try to go out to dinner or to a movie while someone else takes care of the baby.

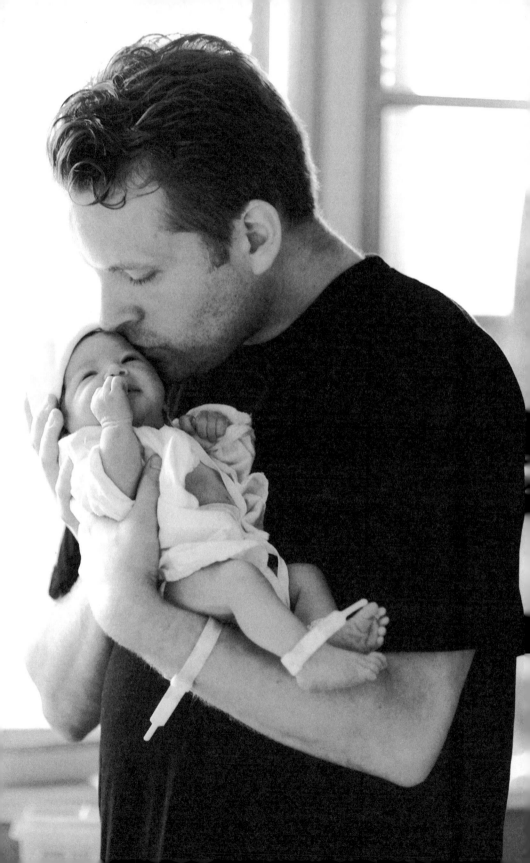

Chapter 7
TIPS FROM THE EXPERTS:
Dads' Birth Stories

ere are some stories from dads who supported their partners through c-sections, twin births, long labors, births with epidurals, and unmedicated births.

JERRY AND NATALIE—
Unmedicated Vaginal Birth

> "She will be going through the most pain she will **ever** experience. She is going to doubt her abilities often, and you as her man need to be there to tell her she is the best and that you can't believe how strong she is."

Natalie went into labor around 3:00 A.M. on April 19. The contractions were a minute on and a minute off when she woke me up about 3:30, saying it was time to go. We had everything in the car already but, of course, I forgot my wallet, so we had to turn around and grab it because I didn't want to be hassled once we got to the hospital. We got to the hospital, and they checked her vitals and everything and then determined they would admit her. We asked for a midwife as soon as we were admitted [the hospital they delivered at allows women to request doctors or midwives for the delivery, no matter who they've been seeing in prenatals, as it's unlikely they'll get the care provider they've been attending prenatals with], and once we were in a room a nurse came by and checked Natalie out. Then the midwife came in and introduced herself.

Natalie wanted very badly to give birth naturally, and that is exactly what she did. She kept saying it hurt and she didn't think she could do it, but everyone, including me, just kept telling her that she could do it and was doing it. As each contraction came, I kept her as comfortable as possible with ice chips, cold compresses, water, massage, encouraging words, and reminders that she would have her baby boy soon. I brushed out her hair, because it was a mess. I massaged her back a little, too, because she had a lot of back labor; the baby came out sunny-side up.

Once he was born there was some meconium, so after placing him on her chest for a few moments they took him over to the warming table, cleared his airways, and monitored him to make sure he hadn't swallowed any. When they started tests for responsiveness, he was not cooperative; he did not cry at all and was very Gumby-like at first. Once he pinked up, the staff were happier, but even when they did the heel prick he did not cry. This concerned the staff, but he ended up crying a good amount once they gave him a bath. I thought it was hilarious: They made him bleed, and he didn't even sniffle, but they put some warm soapy water on him, and he had had enough.

During the birth, I continually told Natalie that I was proud of her and that she was so awesome for doing this without any interventions. When she would doubt herself, I would tell her not to—that she was doing it, so there was no room for "I don't think I can."

I did make one mistake: Natalie yelled at me for texting during the birth. I told the nurse I was telling my wife's brother that his nephew was being born, and the nurse said, "I don't care. Mom can do that. I need you right here right now."

My best advice is to stay off your phone. Have a communications person there to talk to people and relay information so you are 100 percent focused on your wife. It is all about her at this point, and your greatest role is her support.

After all was said and done, Natalie apologized for being short with me and thanked me over and over for being such a great help. She tells everyone that I did good.

BOB AND JENNIFER—
Vaginal Birth with an Epidural

> "Be prepared to be bombarded by friends and family who want to see the baby. Just keep in mind that your partner's recovery is very important, so you might have to put off seeing some people until a few weeks after the birth."

Our baby's birth was much less dramatic than I expected. You have all of these expectations and images derived from movies and television, but in the end it's just a few people in a hospital room. There is no background music, no lighting or special effects or well-quipped one-liners. Aside from the intense emotions, the process was similar to any other hospital or doctor's office visit. Your partner just follows the nurses' instructions and asks for help when she needs it.

Jennifer didn't want to use any pain medications, but she was having back labor, so she ended up getting an epidural. That went smoothly, and everything after that went pretty much to plan. Once she started the pushing process, time just flew by. She pushed for a little over one hour, but it seemed like only a few minutes. It was kind of surreal.

I think that a couple of things helped Jennifer during the birth. Having family in the room with her was really important to her. I was kind of reluctant to have Jennifer's mom and sister in the room during the birth, but in hindsight they really helped to keep her calm. I think what helped her the most during the birth was having a midwife she could trust. I could tell that she really bonded with the midwife, and that bond helped her to relax and concentrate on the birthing process.

After the birth, I stayed with Jennifer at the hospital until she and the baby were released. I tried to do everything I could to accommodate her. I picked up her prescriptions, served her drinks, filled out paperwork, changed the baby's diapers, and did everything else I could to help her to relax so she could recover.

I do wish I'd been a little more cheerful after the birth. Jennifer had gone into labor in the late afternoon. By the time she'd had the baby the next day, I was exhausted from going without sleep. I wish I would have been more upbeat when our families came to visit, but by then I just wanted to be left alone with Jennifer and our new baby.

The most important things to remember are to be supportive of your partner and to let the medical professionals do their jobs. You don't need to get caught up in the technical aspects. Just support your partner and enjoy what will be one of the most memorable moments in your lifetime.

"COBRA" AND SARAH—
Urgent C-Section After Routine Testing

> "Know that your job is to support, not fix. In addition, as a
> friend told me his father-in-law told him, for a while you're
> not even the second fiddle. Be prepared to deal with that,
> and do it well, because your child and his or her mother need
> you more than you need to feel important. Trust that your
> role makes you crucial."

We wanted a natural childbirth, and I figured that we'd done everything right, so in some way I thought we deserved it. I don't normally think like that. When it came to the actual birthing, I expected to really stress out, and to do only an adequate to sub-par job. Truly, I knew I'd read enough, and I'd been active enough in the birthing class. But I figured, with all my fears and anxieties getting in the way, I'd find some way to flub up and be only marginally effective. I'd be disappointing to myself and Sarah.

What actually happened was far different. Sarah went in for routine testing. Since our baby boy seemed small, and his fluid levels were low from time to time, she had to do this weekly, if not twice a week. We'd just acquiesced to a planned c-section on December 14 because of this.

On December 4, Sarah called me, crying, and told me that our son, Bill, was probably going to be born that day. I left work immediately, but once I got to the hospital I found it was a hurry-up-and-wait situation. After making sure Sarah was okay, I went down to the car to get something to read and my laptop. By the time I came back up, Bill's constant monitoring had picked up a drop in heart rate for a few minutes. The staff had decided to do a c-section that wasn't quite an emergency but not quite planned, either. I felt bad that I hadn't been present when they told

Sarah that Bill had bought himself a c-section. She had had to deal with that news alone, while I was on my way upstairs, because I'd wanted a book and my computer, since we thought we were just waiting and watching for four hours. I really wish I'd been there to hold her hand.

So, we had what I call an urgent c-section. Our surgeon was somewhat dismissive of Sarah's fears. I didn't like that one bit. But she was an awesome surgeon. There's a reason doctors become surgeons. I had a son eleven years prior to this who didn't make it since he was born so early, so I had all kinds of fears going through my head. They told me to wait outside the operating room for a few minutes while they prepared my wife for the surgery. I was chomping at the bit to go in, as I knew that Sarah had never been through this before. And, since she was strapped down to a table, unable to see what was happening to her, I knew she'd be scared—especially given the lead-up to the c-section. They let me in after what felt like an eternity.

When I got in there, I swallowed every bit of fear I had and rushed to her side. I was there entirely for her. I told her that it was her show, since she was the one on the table, and that if she wanted me to go with Bill once they pulled him out, that was fine, but I would stay with her until she told me to go.

He was breech, and especially long-armed. And a redhead. I joked that this proved who the father was, but who was the mother? I made several other jokes, too—my natural approach to any situation. Not that many were funny to Sarah, as was also normal for all situations. But the docs loved it.

When they told me I could stand up to see him, Bill was covered in vernix. And he was blue. And bloody. And pretty quiet. He gurgled, but made no real cry. He tried to cry, but the fluid in his mouth prevented him from doing so. The nurses and docs whisked him away to the warmer outside the room. Sarah told me to go with him. So I did.

My friend was there with a video camera. I came close to crying a couple of times as they put an oxygen mask on Bill and worked on warming him. Since I'd already lost a redheaded son, I had a nagging "not again" feeling. But when they said his APGAR score was 7, I stopped worrying.

They took a few minutes to determine whether he needed a trip to the NICU. He was 25 grams under the cutoff, but because he scored so well on his APGAR (he got 9 the second time), there was some debate. Eventually he went up to the NICU, but Sarah got to see him for a few minutes before he did. I followed him up, since I was bound and determined to do skin-to-skin contact with him.

The nurses were excellent. They let me play the Beatles' "In My Life" for him as I held him and sang to him. In light of the fact that I'd never gotten to hold my first son until the day he died, this felt like a very important moment to me, but it seems even more so in retrospect. My main goal was to warm up my boy so that he could keep his own body heat. It worked. He had to stay only a couple of hours. Then we went down to Sarah, so that she could feed him in the recovery room. From then on, we've had him in our care.

Sarah has often said that she's had complete and total confidence in my ability to care for our son. I keep saying that this is unfounded, but I also refuse to shake that confidence. Now that I think about it, I've been there in my son's life continuously since the moment he was pulled out. In retrospect, again, that holds even more significance because I couldn't do anything for my first son.

Because Sarah had had a c-section, I did a lot of the getting-up-and-getting-Bill when he cried in the hospital. I held him a lot at night so that she'd get to sleep more. I coordinated people bringing us food and visiting. I also made sure we watched the idiotic videos they insisted we watch. I was a good advocate with the nurses and doctors for Sarah's needs. I made sure that Sarah advocated for herself, and I bolstered her when she was overwhelmed. Since I'm awful with paperwork, I was surprised quite a bit that I was able to take care of all his birth certificate and Social Security stuff. I also washed Sarah's feet in the shower, getting soaked in the process.

The night before Sarah and Bill came home, when I'd not slept in almost a day, I went home and cleaned the house completely—top to bottom—so that Sarah and Bill came home to a good, clean home. I then drove back to the hospital with all of the stuff Sarah needed.

When we got home, I did anything and everything around the house so that all she had to do was take care of Bill. I took two weeks off of work—which became four weeks, since I'm a teacher and winter break came. I did all the laundry, dishes, cooking, cleaning, dog care, and networking with people wanting to visit. I woke up with Bill, changed him a lot, and prepped him for Sarah's breastfeeding. I also drove us everywhere we needed to go. When we went to the doctor, I made sure we had all the necessary paperwork (again, no mean feat for me), and bag full o' stuff that is suddenly necessary with a baby.

My best advice is to do what the mother expects you to do, even if you don't want to do it. My wife and I were very clear about how we'd handle hypothetical situations, which was especially important given the fact that several happened. Because I knew very clearly what Sarah wanted me to do regarding Bill in the NICU, and she knew my comfort levels, we were able to operate almost seamlessly in caring for Bill. Also, I knew exactly how she wanted me to support her, and what I needed to let her do on her own.

My wife is amazing. I don't know how I won the lottery when it comes to wives, but I am so glad that I did. My son couldn't ask for a better mom, and it's really nice to know that I'm the support for someone so awesome. It makes being the third fiddle more than fulfilling.

AMY AND STEVE—Unmedicated Vaginal Birth

"Birth hurts, but God gave women the strength and body
to do it."

Amy went into labor in the morning while I was at work. By the time she called me to come home and we got to the hospital, she was already 6 centimeters dilated. I encouraged her. I knew our birth plan and the things she wanted. We danced, we got in the shower, and we tried a lot of different positions. Our childbirth class had given me valuable information and helped me do my very best. Her labor moved fast, but she did a great job. Amy stayed calm and focused. Five hours later our baby boy was born.

After our baby was born, I continued to give encouragement. I did anything I could do to make her feel more comfortable and happy. We learned that the hospital and all the nurses could be overwhelming, so we walked around. I would hold and spend quiet time bonding with the baby so my wife could sleep or shower.

Amy had a natural birth, without drugs, and she did great. It was a lot nicer this way, and she felt like herself afterward. My best advice is to weigh all the options and the pro and cons of using drugs. Make sure you give lots of encouragement, so that you and your partner have the best birth experience you can.

JON AND BETH—Vaginal Birth with a Long Prodomal Labor and an Epidural

> "My advice to dads is to take care of yourself so you can take care of others. And have an alternate coach, or more than one."

Everyone told us to have a birth plan, but to be prepared to abandon it—sage advice, indeed. We stuck to our birth plan, avoiding medication, perhaps a little longer than made sense, but abandoning it earlier might have left us feeling less satisfied. We used all the comfort techniques we had learned, and then adjusted the plan as circumstances changed. But after fifty-five hours of natural labor, we needed some interventions. What I mostly remember was how powerless I felt during the long labor. Fortunately, Beth's parents and mine were around to take shifts. I needed sleep to be at my best when active labor arrived, as I feel I was.

For the eventual decision to go with Pitocin and the epidural, I took comfort from, and relied heavily on, the advice of friends and family who had recently been through the process. Beth needed sleep badly, which the epidural permitted. Pitocin moved the process along.

My memories of active labor are a little hazier. I remember doing lots of hand-holding, providing lots of emotional support, and assuring her that she could in fact do this, that she had the strength. I was surprised by my physical role at the end; I hadn't realized that I would be holding this and pushing that with much of my weight, though I'm thrilled to have taken such an active role.

After the baby was born, I feel I failed miserably in the hospital. Our son was sent to the NICU, and I stayed there as much as I could, to the point of exhaustion, and then slept. Since what he mostly needed was food, I couldn't help much. I was able to help Beth with her latch. And I brought her sushi.

TED AND JESSICA—Vaginal Births with Complications Afterward

> "Hold her hand, tell her how great she is doing, and, if a complication surfaces, stay calm so your wife stays calm. Let her know she is going to be okay and everything is going to be fine."

Both of our daughters' actual births were fine, but there were complications afterward. After the first birth, Jessica got really dizzy and pale. She turned white as a ghost. No one really knows what happened. They think a piece of the placenta came off or there was a hemorrhage. She was okay after about fifteen minutes. With the second birth, things were worse. At the same point in the process, she had clotting inside her uterus. The doctor reached his hand inside the uterus and kept pulling out clot after clot. Jessica lost a lot of blood and came really close to having emergency surgery. She needed blood transfusions and took almost three months to fully recover.

During each birth I did all I could to keep her calm and to let her know the baby was okay. I too stayed calm, even though I was scared, so I didn't make her more scared than she already was. I held her hand and was by her side the whole time.

I did get frustrated with the doctors at the second birth. I told them what had happened after the first birth, when Jessica got a little sick and pale. But when the head doctor came in at the end of the second birth, once Jessica was okay, he said, "How come nobody told us about the complications in the past birth?" I almost came unglued.

After both births Jessica needed a lot of rest. She made the decision not to breastfeed, as she was just too weak. So I gave our daughters their bottles and changed them while Jessica rested in the hospital and at home until she was able to get her strength back.

The best advice I would give to dads is to stay calm and remember that your wife comes first. Hold her hand, tell her how great she is doing, and, if a complication surfaces, stay calm so your wife stays calm. Let her know that she is going to be okay and everything is going to be fine. Make sure you are by her side the entire time.

MICHELLE AND RYAN—Twin C-section Birth

"Pay attention to your partner. Put your phone away, and just be there for your partner."

My partner went into labor about six weeks before our kids were born—twins!—so we had a couple trips to the hospital, initially with fingers crossed that they wouldn't come but eventually excited to think it could be the actual day. The weeks before the birth were hard, because Michelle was on a medication that she had to take around the clock—alarms went off all night—and she wasn't supposed to be up moving around much.

On "The Day," she went into labor in the morning, and we made our way to the hospital. She wanted to go unmedicated and to be in the shower and walking the halls, but her doctor wouldn't let her get out of bed. That made contractions a lot harder on her and changed our birth plan. When they broke her water bag, it had a funny smell, and it grossed me out. That evening, she was stuck at 8 centimeters dilated for four hours, and one of our sons wasn't doing so well, so we ended up going for a c-section. The kids were born around 5:45 P.M. and then spent ten days in the NICU due to a strep-B infection and their small size.

From my perspective, the birth went fine. Both boys are healthy and happy now. But my partner wanted an unmedicated, vaginal birth, so I don't think she's happy that her labor ended in a c-section.

During the birth, the most helpful thing I did was to be there. And I don't mean just physically, but mentally as well. It's probably a good thing that cell phones were just phones back then; the distractions were so much easier to shut off than they are nowadays. I believe that being there to help her, answer questions, track down people, call family, etc., was the most important role for me.

The biggest mistake I made was to take too much stuff to the hospital. I remember having arms full of things when we went up to the hospital room.

After the boys were born, I was there as much as I could be, walking with her and taking pictures of the kids to her while she was stuck in her bed. After she was discharged from the hospital, I made sure she got rest and ate well at home between trips to the hospital to see the boys.

Birth Jargon Explained

Active labor: The phase of labor when the cervix opens from 4 to 7 centimeters. It begins when contractions become regular and the mom starts to get uncomfortable. She needs a lot of support during this phase (some women yell, curse, or hit, so look out). Most couples wait until active labor begins before heading to the birthing facility.

Amnihook: A flat plastic stick with a small hook at the end, used to break the bag of waters (that is, to perform an amniotomy).

Amniotic fluid: Clear, sterile liquid that surrounds, cushions, and protects the baby in the amniotic sac. In late pregnancy, the baby drinks the fluid and then pees it back out.

Amniotic sac: Also called the membranes, this is your baby's home inside the uterus. Full of amniotic fluid and the baby, the sac is a thick membrane that grows out of the placenta and protects the baby from bacteria. You may see the amniotic sac attached to the placenta when the placenta comes out. The sac looks something like a cloudy plastic bag.

Amniotomy: The rupture of the amniotic sac (or bag of waters, or membranes) with an amnihook. Like popping a balloon, this procedure is also called AROM, for artificial rupture of the membranes. See page 110 for advice on supporting your partner through an amniotomy.

Analgesics: Narcotic medication given to "take the edge off" contractions. In less than five minutes, analgesics can make contractions more manageable and calm a panicking woman. The effect lasts only one to three hours. Potential risks include disorientation, hallucination, drowsiness, and dizziness in moms; the slowing of labor; respiratory problems in the baby (if the analgesics are still in effect at birth), although other medications can counteract this; and a baby's initial lack of interest in breastfeeding.

APGAR: A baby's first test, by which the staff measure on a scale of 0 to 10 how well the baby is adjusting to life. Scores are assigned for the baby's appearance, pulse, grimace or cry (when tapped on the foot or rubbed with a cloth), activity level, and respiration.

Baby blues: Feelings of sadness, anxiety, and irritation after giving birth. Caused by hormonal shifts and sleep deprivation, these feelings are normal during the first two weeks.

Back labor: Pain in a mother's back during contractions, usually caused by a baby's lying in a posterior position, with his head against Mom's spine. This makes for a difficult labor. See page 98 for ways to help.

Bag of waters: Amniotic sac.

Birth plan: A written description of how your partner wants to give birth and how the two of you would like your newborn cared for at the birthing facility. The birth plan should be designed to eliminate miscommunication and help save you from repeating yourself over and over and over and. . . .

Birthing ball: A big ball women use to get into comfortable positions during pregnancy and labor. Theresa finds this her most valuable tool in her childbirth classes. It's also called a yoga, exercise, or Pilates ball.

Bloody show: Bloody mucus that comes from the cervix as contractions cause the cervix to soften and open. Your partner might produce some of this all through labor, and it may have a light smell. Though it may give you the heebie-jeebies, a bloody show is normal.

Bonding: Emotional and physical attachment between parents and their children.

Braxton-Hicks: Prelabor contractions, which may or may not start at about twenty weeks' gestation. Just practice for later labor contractions, Braxton-Hicks do not cause the cervix to soften and open. They are usually not painful, though they may be uncomfortable and annoying. Some women are very aware of them, but others aren't.

Breech baby: A baby who is positioned in the womb with her butt or one or both feet pointing down. Babies lying sideways, or transverse, are sometimes called breech as well. In the United States, few doctors or midwives allow women to birth a breech baby vaginally. Most providers will schedule a c-section instead.

Care provider: For the purposes of this book, a midwife, obstetrician, or family-practice doctor.

Cervical ripening agent: Prostaglandins (hormone-like substances) in tablet, gel, or tampon form put on or near the cervix to induce labor before the cervix has naturally softened and thinned. In some women cervical ripening agents start labor, but usually another induction technique follows.

Cervix: The opening of the uterus. Closed, it looks like a pair of puckered lips. During labor, contractions cause the cervix to soften and open so the baby can enter the birth canal. How open the cervix is defines the phase of labor: early, active, or transition. This is what the nurse, midwife, or doctor is feeling for during a vaginal exam.

Cesarean birth: Abdominal surgery used to get the baby out, usually because the provider judges the health of the mother or baby to be at risk. A cesarean poses its own risks: infection, bleeding, and longer healing time for the mother; lower APGAR scores for the baby; and breastfeeding problems.

Childbirth educator: An expert in pregnancy and childbirth who teaches classes. These women are enthusiastic about birth, and some enjoy grossing out dads ("I do not," Theresa says).

Colic: A lot of crying. A baby is said to have colic if he has cried for three hours a day at least three times a week for three weeks.

Contractions: Tightenings of the uterus that start out short and mild and increase to long, regular, painful squeezes, making a mom's belly rock-hard. (This is not the time to remind your partner that she's always wanted rock-hard abs.)

Crowning: The point at which the vagina is completely stretched open by the baby's head.

C-section: Cesarean birth.

Dilation: The opening of the cervix, measured in centimeters by a nurse, midwife, or doctor by the insertion of two fingers into the birth canal. Unless you've had training you shouldn't try checking her dilation for her.

Doula: A person, usually a woman, who helps couples during pregnancy, labor, and the postpartum period. Most are hired privately, though some birthing facilities offer birth doulas, who provide physical, emotional, and informational support during labor. Some birth doulas work only with women planning to give birth naturally (without pain medications); others will work with those planning an epidural or c-section.

Antepartum and postpartum doulas work in the home. An antepartum doula helps during a difficult pregnancy, usually because the mother is on bed rest. A postpartum doula, trained in newborn care and women's postpartum health, helps with minor breastfeeding problems, baby care, errands, and light chores in the weeks after birth. Antepartum and postpartum doulas are like helpful relatives. You have to pay them, but you can tell them what to do, and they won't judge you or make you feel guilty.

See pages 23 and 172 for information about hiring a doula.

Early labor: The phase of labor in which the cervix opens to 4 centimeters and contractions become regular, though they shouldn't be intense yet. Unless labor is being induced or her bag of waters has broken, a woman and her partner usually spend early labor at home.

Effacement: The thinning of the cervix, measured as a percentage: 0 percent is very thick, like the inside of your cheek; 100 percent is very thin, like your eyelid. The cervix has to thin before it can open, or dilate. A nurse, midwife, or doctor can measure effacement in a vaginal exam.

Epidural: A very popular regional "block," in which medication is injected into the epidural space of the spine to take away much of the pain of birth but leave a feeling of pressure, so that—in theory, at least—the woman can still push the baby out. The use of epidurals is a hot topic among pregnant women and birthing professionals; some strongly support their use, and others strongly oppose it. See page 13 for a discussion of the pros and cons.

Episiotomy: A surgical incision made to enlarge the vaginal opening. This procedure is no longer routine, though some doctors perform it much more than others. Generally, an episiotomy is warranted only if the baby has to be born quickly, if forceps are to be used (as they are very uncommonly now in the United States), or if the mother is too exhausted to push the baby out.

Fetal distress: Signs in labor that the baby isn't doing well, such as a change in the heartbeat or the passing of meconium. Fetal distress often requires more monitoring and may result in a c-section.

Fetal monitor: A device that measures the mother's contractions and the baby's heartbeat and graphs them on a strip of paper. Usually, a computer monitor in the nurses' station also displays the graph. There are two types of fetal monitors, internal and external, and monitoring can be either continuous or intermittent. See page 83 for more information.

Focal point: Anything a woman focuses on during contractions—a picture, face, stuffed animal, pattern, or random object in the room. An internal focal point is something she imagines, like a flower or the ocean. See Visualizations.

Foley catheter: A thin, flexible tube usually inserted through the urethra and into the bladder to drain urine, but also sometimes inserted through the cervix and inflated to help induce labor.

Forceps: Two metal tongs that fit around a baby's head so the doctor can pull the baby out. Forceps are used infrequently in the United States, and usually only in emergencies.

Gestational diabetes: High blood sugar in the mother during pregnancy. If your partner has this, she'll have to modify her diet, and she may have to take insulin. Untreated, gestational diabetes can make a baby grow too big to fit through the mom's pelvis, and this increases the chances of an induction and a c-section.

Induction: Medical intervention to get labor started. Induction may involve the use of a cervical ripening agent, a Foley catheter, an amniotomy, Pitocin, or a combination of these. Inductions are generally done for medical reasons or "going postdate"—that is, beyond forty-two weeks' gestation. An induction increases the odds of a c-section, because the mother's body is forced into labor before it's ready, and also the odds of an epidural, because induced labors are often more difficult.

Intravenous (IV) drip: A plastic bag of liquids, which may include medication, that hangs from a pole and is connected to a tube that's inserted into a vein in a woman's hand or arm. The fluid drips into her vein. Many birthing facilities require that every woman in labor have an IV, or at least a saline lock, just in case she needs medications later.

Labor positions: Positions that can help relieve the pain of contractions and prompt the cervix to open and the baby to drop down into the birth canal. These positions include sitting on a birthing ball or backward on a chair, lunging, squatting, kneeling while leaning forward, and resting on all fours. Childbirth classes give couples a chance to try the various positions, and doulas, nurses, and midwives may suggest one or another during labor.

Lactation consultant: An expert who helps women with breastfeeding problems. To earn her certification, she must take classes and pass a very difficult test. Some lactation consultants work in hospitals, where they help women get started with breastfeeding, and others are available for hire privately. Visit ILCA.org to find a lactation consultant in your area.

Lochia: Bloody vaginal discharge after a woman gives birth. It begins immediately after the birth and is very heavy for a day or two. Then it darkens and tapers off over the next four to six weeks. Most women wear menstrual pads for the first few weeks after giving birth.

Meconium: Baby's first bowel movement, with a blackish-greenish color. Some babies pass meconium before birth (see page 111).

Membranes: Also called the bag of waters (see Amniotic sac).

Midwife: A childbirth specialist who monitors pregnancies, attends births, and handles some birth emergencies but refers clients to an obstetrician if surgery becomes necessary. A midwife may or may not have nursing or other medical credentials. She may attend home births, hospital births, or both. Certification of midwives varies from state to state.

Mucus plug: A big clump of mucus from the cervix that a woman loses in prelabor or early labor. Losing the mucus plug indicates that labor will begin soon, within hours, days, or weeks.

Natural childbirth: Depending on who is using it, this term can refer to any vaginal birth, a birth without an epidural or analgesics, or a birth without any sort of medical intervention, including an IV.

Neonatal Intensive-Care Unit (NICU): An intensive-care unit for newborns, equipped with everything a struggling baby might need.

Newborn procedures: Routine treatments performed on a baby after birth. They include the placement of erythromycin ointment in the eyes, to help prevent an infection; a shot of vitamin K, to promote blood clotting; a visual and tactile exam; weighing; measuring of body length; and the sampling of blood for genetic screening tests. You can delay these procedures until the baby is a few hours old, and you may refuse some of them if you choose, even if they are required by state law. Discuss the pros and cons with your partner and her doctor or midwife, and consider writing your preferences into the birth plan.

Obstetrician-gynecologist (OB-GYN): A surgeon trained in gynecological health who has additional training in high-risk deliveries. Most U.S. births are attended by obstetricians.

Oxytocin: The main hormone involved with labor and birth. It causes the uterus to contract. It's also the "cuddle hormone" or "love hormone" that humans produce when they fall in love and when they meet their babies for the first time.

Perineal massage: A massage technique that may prevent perineal tearing. During perineal massage, a finger is lightly inserted into the vagina and rubbed back and forth along the perineum. Some women have their partners start doing this weeks before labor starts; others have it done only by the nurse, midwife, or doctor during pushing. If your partner wants to try it ahead of time, use a good lubricant, and be gentle. You might think of it as foreplay.

Perineal tearing: Tearing in the perineum that occurs as the baby is born. Most tears are from the vagina toward the rectum, though some are toward the urethra.

Perineum: The area between the rectum and the birth canal.

Pitocin: A synthetic form of the hormone oxytocin administered intravenously to induce or augment labor contractions. Pitocin may also be given after birth, to assist in the delivery of the placenta or to stop or prevent a hemorrhage. You might discuss pros and cons with your partner's care provider.

Placenta: An organ that develops in the uterus during pregnancy to provide the baby with nutrients and eliminate waste products. It remains attached to the inside wall of the uterus until the baby is born. After a woman gives birth to a baby, she gives birth to the placenta, which is sometimes called the afterbirth.

Postpartum depression: Depression occurring in a mother or father after a baby is born. Symptoms include feeling detached from the baby; feeling sad, irritated, or anxious; having headaches, backaches, or stomachaches with no apparent cause; and sleeping or eating problems. Please seek help if you or your partner has these symptoms.

Postpartum psychosis: A rare form of postpartum depression in which a woman hears voices that aren't real, experiences irrational fears, and exhibits odd behavior. It may be hard to imagine a woman convinced that aliens will kidnap her baby, but a psychotic mom might hurt or kill herself, her baby, or other family members. She needs professional help immediately.

Prelabor: A period of mild warm-up contractions (Braxton-Hicks) leading up to the big day. During prelabor, which can last for weeks, a woman may often think she's in labor, only to have her contractions fizzle out. The cervix often starts opening during prelabor, although the mom isn't technically in labor yet.

Prodomal labor: Labor with strong, rhythmic, and painful contractions but little or no cervical change. This labor pattern can last for days or weeks, and it is very challenging for moms and their partners. No one is sure why some women experience prodomal labor.

Rooming in: Keeping the baby in the mother's hospital room. This practice is highly endorsed by the American Academy of Pediatrics.

Saline lock: A cap on the end of a tube in a vein, for quick connection to an intravenous (IV) line. This allows mobility for a woman who doesn't currently need an IV. Most hospitals require laboring women to have a saline lock even if they're planning an unmedicated birth.

Skin-to-skin contact: Cuddling a bare-chested baby against an adult's bare chest. This helps keep the baby warm and calm; helps stabilize her heart rate, respiration, and blood glucose levels; and promotes bonding and breastfeeding. Skin-to-skin contact provides benefits throughout the baby's first year.

Station: The measurement of the baby's descent through the pelvis, measured in relation to two pelvic bones, the ischial spines. Station is measured from -4 to +4. At -4, the baby is high in the pelvis; at +4, the baby is nearly born. Positive numbers show good progress.

Strep B: Also called group B strep, group B streptococcus, or GBS, these bacteria live on our skin and in some women's vaginas. Occasionally, a baby can acquire a strep B infection while passing through the birth canal, and this can make the baby very sick. For this reason, providers test women for strep B at about thirty-six weeks' gestation. Women who test positive are given intravenous antibiotics every four hours during labor.

Stripping the membranes: A procedure in which a doctor or midwife pulls the amniotic sac away from the cervix and stretches the cervix with her fingers. Also called sweeping the membranes, this is done in an attempt to get labor started. It may work if the mother is close enough to starting labor naturally.

Transition: The hardest part of labor, but usually the shortest. During this phase, in which the cervix opens from 7 to 10 centimeters, the contractions are intense, long, and close together. Mom may be cranky and demanding, and she may feel sick. She may shake, sweat, and vomit.

Umbilical cord: A thick cord extending from the baby to the placenta. Until birth, the baby gets all her nutrients and oxygen through this cord.

Uterus: A muscle that surrounds and stretches with the baby and contracts to get the baby out. Also called the womb.

Vacuum cap: An obstetric suction cup that's applied to a baby's head to assist in delivery. It's connected to a pump that looks like a Shop Vac. Vacuum extraction is done when a baby needs to be born in a hurry or when the mother is too exhausted to continue pushing.

Vaginal birth after cesarean (VBAC): Vaginal birth to a woman who has had one or more babies by cesarean in the past.

Visualization: A woman's intentional imagining of a place, thing, or sequence of events to help her relax during contractions. Common subjects include the ocean and flowers. Some visualizations involve scripts to read or listen to. A visualization can be a form of hypnosis.

Waters. Amniotic fluid. A woman's "waters break" when the amniotic sac ruptures spontaneously.

Helpful Organizations and Websites

American Academy of Pediatrics (AAP): An association of over sixty thousand pediatricians, or doctors who specialize in caring for children. The AAP does a lot of research and, based on that research, provides recommendations for American pediatricians. See AAP.org for more information.

Birthing from Within: Pam England's book by the same title spawned classes based on her theory of birth as a rite of passage. Birthing from Within classes emphasize natural, unmedicated birth and include art and journaling. Go to BirthingFromWithin.com for more information or to find a local class.

Bradley Method: Also called husband-coached childbirth, this approach was designed by Dr. Robert Bradley for couples aiming for a natural, unmedicated birth. The classes go into depth about breathing, massage, and other comfort techniques. Go to BradleyBirth.com for more information.

Childbirth International: This organization provides home-study courses and certification for childbirth educators, doulas, and breastfeeding counselors. ChildbirthInternational.com has a worldwide search service for these professionals.

DONA International: The largest doula association in the world, DONA trains and certifies antepartum, birth, and postpartum doulas. DONA.org provides a doula-finder service and a lot of information about doulas, childbirth, and the postpartum experience.

HypnoBirthing and Hypnobabies: These are two separate companies offering similar childbirth-preparation courses. Moms are taught relaxation techniques similar to hypnosis. The companies claim that mothers who complete their programs and apply what they learn give birth without pain. Theresa has worked with several couples who have used HypnoBirthing; the moms gave birth without medication but did experience some discomfort. Go to HypnoBirthing.com and Hypnobabies.com for more information or to find a local practitioner.

International Childbirth Education Association (ICEA): This non-profit organization trains childbirth educators and doulas in a philosophy of family-centered maternity and newborn care, which respects parents' right to make decisions based on knowledge of alternatives. A members' directory is available at ICEA.org.

International Lactation Consultant Association (ILCA): This international organization certifies lactation consultants and establishes their standards of practice. You can find a local ILCA member at ILCA.org.

La Leche League International: This organization provides information for breastfeeding mothers through chapters all over the world. Run by volunteer lactation counselors, most chapters provide weekly meetings at which breastfeeding mothers can talk together and get breastfeeding assistance. Go to LLLI.org to find a local chapter.

Lamaze International: A nonprofit organization that certifies childbirth educators, many of whom work for hospitals, and promotes "a natural, healthy, and safe approach to pregnancy, childbirth, and early parenting." Visit Lamaze.org to locate a Lamaze childbirth class, read an online magazine on pregnancy and birth, watch birth videos, sign up for a weekly pregnancy newsletter, or join in the Ask an Expert Forum.

National Center for Fathering: This website offers newsletters, articles, and podcasts for all fathers in all walks of life. Go to Fathers.com for more information.

Index